Nursing Care for the Dying Patient and the Family

Nursing Care for the Dying Patient and the Family

Winifred Hector, MPhil RNT

and

Sarah Whitfield, MSc BSc(Hons) SRN

William Heinemann Medical Books Ltd
London

First published 1982

© Winifred Hector and Sarah Whitfield, 1982

ISBN 0-433-14219-7

Typeset by Inforum Ltd, Portsmouth
Printed in Great Britain by Redwood Burn Ltd,
Trowbridge, Wiltshire

Contents

what we now offer to others. There are many we cannot name who have contributed their views and experiences. The stories related are based on real life, but names and localities have been altered.

Nurses are commonly written about in the feminine, since women are in the majority and it is cumbersome to try to allude to both sexes. The work of men in the field of terminal care is gratefully acknowledged. Where the patient's sex is not material we have used the masculine gender and hope this literary device is not offensive.

Every nurse owes a debt to Dame Cicely Saunders for her practical skill, sympathy and pioneering work in the care of the dying, and for her willingness to share her knowledge with others. Sister Paula and the doctors and nurses of St Joseph's Hospice, Mare Street, London E8, are especially thanked for their kindness to one of us during professional collaboration, and for the marvellous standard of care they provide. St Ann's Hospice, Heald Green, Manchester, provided experience and counselling for the other author, and are remembered gratefully. Dr Jean Kay, St Barnabas' Home, Worthing, is thanked for practical advice and information. Miss J. A. Clark, formerly a paediatric sister of St Bartholomew's Hospital has wide experience and understanding of children dying of cancer, and of their parents, and made this available to us. Joan Matthias typed the manuscript with her usual efficiency, and offered helpful suggestions.

Owen Evans, formerly of Heinemann Medical Books Ltd, encouraged us to write this, and to him and to the present staff, we offer thanks.

W. E. H.
S. A. W.

Preface

In October 1347 merchant ships coming from the Black Sea put into Messina in Sicily with dead and dying men at the oars. The Black Death had arrived in Europe from the Far East and no one knows how many millions died. People thought it must be the end of the world. From time to time outbreaks of plague returned; that in London in 1666 was only the worst of many.

In such calamities care of the dying can only be minimal; even disposal of the dead may be hard. Even today we may be overwhelmed by the magnitude of the problems that may confront us. Catastrophes like earthquakes and famine happen, in which doctors and nurses have to do what they can to reduce human suffering. Every century brings its own problems; today we have aeroplane crashes in which hundreds die.

In thinking about all these manifold aspects of death, it became necessary for the authors to define their objectives, and this book is for those of us who have to see our individual patients through their last illness or injury, and to help their families. Psychologists and sociologists have paid much attention to the mechanisms of grief and bereavement, but nurses ask themselves and their colleagues and teachers 'What should I do?', 'What shall I say?', 'Did I do rightly or wrongly?' It is this kind of need for practical information and comfort that we would like to try to meet.

We have both learned from our colleagues and patients

1

Views on death

When planning for or writing about the care of the dying, it must not be forgotten that what we say will only apply to the present, and to a developed society with certain social beliefs and medical skills. Were we writing this a century ago, in Victorian times, we would be dealing with an era in which most deaths took place at home, when there were many deaths among babies and children, when many diseases were fatal which are now curable, and their effects were ascribed to God's will. Children had a vivid awareness of death, and saw it often among playmates and siblings. Sankey and Moody's Hymnbook, so much used at the turn of the century, is full of insights into the popular and rather matter of fact views of death.

> 'I should like to die', said Willy,
> 'If my papa could die too.
> But he says he isn't ready,
> Cos he's got so much to do'.

Were we to look at beliefs and burial rituals in other parts of the world today, we would find great disparity of ideas and practices. One of the things we know best about very early times is the way in which the dead were buried, and we can deduce in many cases the views about life after death. In the barrows of Stone Age man, and in the Pyramids of the Egyptian Pharaohs are found goods for use in the after-life. These may be modest provisions for eating, drinking and hunting, or lavish expenditure of treasure, and in some cultures of slaves and wives to wait on the dead in the other world.

Ancestor worship is widespread in the Far East, but just as common is fear of the dead, who are thought to be a danger to the living. Only last century in this country suicides were buried not in consecrated ground, but at crossroads. There are tribes in which a dead man is taken out not through the door, lest he find his way back, but by breaking down the wall.

There are great occasions in human life — birth, puberty, and death — which are accompanied, even in sophisticated communities, by rites and ceremonies. While these tend to diminish somewhat with time, they are meant to ensure safety and good fortune, and can be of great reassurance. Thus mourning, funeral, flowers, obituaries, wakes and memorial services help relatives to express grief, and to make them feel that the departed has been ensured a kind of after life, either in people's memories, or in a more formal sense if religion prescribes it.

These rituals may be of immediate concern to the nurse whose patient has died, and of more distant concern too if we accept that the caring community will want to ensure the emotional welfare of the family after the death.

The way in which the last rites are conducted in any community is influenced by many factors; the following are some of the most important.

1. *Religion*. In some a greater emphasis is placed on life after death than in others. Some prescribe the way in which the body is dealt with, e.g. by burial or cremation.

2. *Climate*. Rapid disposal of remains is necessary in hot regions, where cremation is common.

3. *Mortality rates*. Where death is common, attitudes are different from those in countries or times where expectation of life is high, and death of a patient may be seen as a kind of defeat for doctors and nurses.

4. *Social attitudes and customs*. In the United States, which

might be thought similar to Great Britain in so many ways, embalming is almost universal, and the custom of 'viewing' the departed with the family by friends is common.

When someone dies at home, he may remain in his home until his funeral, and this is the usual practice in rural areas and closeknit communities. In others, he is taken to a funeral parlour after death. Older people in the country still retain a matter-of-fact attitude about their own death, and may have clean night clothes ready in which to be 'put forth' for burial.

5. *The model of the medical and nursing role* is changed with time. Doctors and nurses now have better methods of easing the transition from life to death, and in general a wider view of their responsibilities to the family, and a desire to alleviate grief and offer support. These opportunities and roles are the same for all patients, but often the religious and cultural beliefs of the patient and his family are of great importance in deciding the attitude and duties of the nurse. The section that follows is a brief account of some of the tenets of the great religions which the nurse should know. It is in no sense a definitive description, but a selection of some aspects which are relevant to us as nurses.

Religious Teaching

Christians are united in believing that there is life after death, expressed in some creeds as belief in 'the resurrection of the body'. This means not that the actual physical body that was used in life is to be resumed, but that more is implied than an impersonal thin kind of survival.

Roman Catholics

The Roman Catholic Church has the most precisely expressed sets of beliefs and practices, but recently there has been a tendency to modify these, mostly by change in emphasis rather than in doctrine. Catholics believe that the life hereafter is influenced by the way we live here, and they hope to follow the teaching of their church, and when they fail, to confess their failure to the priest, and receive absolution.

A Catholic who knows himself to be very ill would wish to

make his confession, receive absolution, and if he is able, the Sacrament. Anointing with holy oil used to be known as Extreme Unction, and was used for those thought to be dying. This rite is now called Anointing of the Sick, and its use is not confined to those at the point of death.

Nurses are aware that if patients are asked what their religion is, some will reply that they are Catholic, but a 'bad' one. They mean that they have stopped going to Mass. These people when sick or gravely ill may or may not wish to speak to a priest; they should be given the opportunity, which most seem to take, but not pressed.

Until quite recently all Roman Catholics were buried, as Jesus Christ was, but cremation has now been made permissible, and there are prescribed rites for it. Donation of eyes, kidneys or other organs for replacement surgery is allowed. Normal last offices are used. The parish priest is usually a friend of the family, and takes an active part in comforting them and supporting them.

Baptism into the Catholic church is an essential rite for the children of Catholic parents. If an unbaptised infant or a newly born baby seems likely to die, the mother should be told and the priest called. If he does not arrive in time, a lay person, not necessarily a Catholic, may perform the rite, by pouring water on the baby's head, and saying, 'I baptize you in the name of the Father, the Son, and the Holy Ghost'. If the child is stillborn, conditional baptism can be given. Pouring the water, the nurse says, 'If you are able to be baptised, I baptise you. . . . The priest is told what has happened, and proceeds as he thinks fit.

The Anglican Communion

The Church of England has no official rite of Extreme Unction, but provides for confession to a priest by those who feel the need, and the administration of the Holy Eucharist to the sick and dying. The Church of England contains within it people who place differing emphasis on different parts of its teaching. Some find their greatest comfort in its sacraments, others in Bible reading and prayer. There is provision for the anointing of the sick.

Church of England prayer books and services have been

and still are undergoing revision, mostly in the direction of rendering them into English more easily understood than the magnificent if sometimes obscure 1662 version. There are no official views on the disposal of the body, or against post-mortem examination.

Non-Conformists

Members of the Free Churches do not differ from other Christians in looking with hope to a life after death. They contain within their ranks people with differing views about the ultimate destination of the dead, but they place more stress on the mercy of God than on rites such as anointing for the dying.

The minister would always wish to be called if a member of his faith were dying, knowing that his experience and his professional training will help him to support and comfort the family. He sees his role as that of the caring and concerned friend of patient and relatives rather than a bringer of sacraments.

Jews

The majority of the half a million Jews in this country live in the Greater London area, and most of the others in the big cities like Manchester.

What distinguished the Jews when they were establishing their identity three thousand years ago was their belief that their God was the unique and only one, among the many gods of the Middle East, and their detailed dietary and hygienic laws, which presumably gave them a survival advantage over neighbouring tribes. Orthodox Jews still maintain not only their religious beliefs, but adhere scrupulously to the dietary rules and the total life style prescribed. Their diet must consist of kosher food. Meat must have been drained of all blood, so must have come from a Jewish slaughterhouse. The flesh of the pig in any form is absolutely forbidden. Milk and meat are not eaten at the same meal, or cooked in the same saucepans or with the same utensils. A hospital or hospice would not be able to keep such rules for Orthodox Jewish patients, but a kosher diet can be supplied by a catering firm.

Reformed or Liberal Jews, while still thinking of themselves as Jewish in every sense, and attending synagogue, have adopted more relaxed views on diet, and will eat ordinary food prepared by Gentiles, though many of them do not like pork or bacon.

Jews have warm family attachments, and the dying patient will usually have his relatives around him, and the rabbi may be present to recite the traditional prayers. 'Hear O Israel, the Lord our God is one' is the last prayer, expressing the core of the Jewish faith in the uniqueness of Jehovah. The way in which the Jew is treated after death in hospital will vary from one place to another. The family may wish to prepare the body for burial, or a Gentile nurse may perform last offices in the usual way. Some Jews do not want the body of a believer to be directly handled by a Gentile, and it may be a hospital practice that the nurse puts on disposable gloves, and wraps the body in a sheet ready for transfer to the mortuary, and relatives inform their own undertaker.

Lamentation, weeping, and overt expression of grief by the relatives is normal, and if possible the Jew should be in a sideroom so that free expression of emotion is possible without upsetting other patients in an open ward.

If the Jew dies at home, he will be wrapped in a sheet, laid on the floor with the feet towards the door, and a lighted candle placed at his head. The Burial Society of the Synagogue, when informed of a death, will carry out the last ritual washing and clothing of the body ready for interment. Traditionally, the body is not left unattended until the burial. Jews do not allow embalming or cremation and early burial is practised. Post-mortem examination is not permitted, unless it is ordered by the civil authority, but if a Jew expressly desires that organs be given after his death for replacement surgery, his wishes are respected. Burial is not permitted on the Sabbath Day.

Jews believe in eternal life, and the twenty-third psalm is as beloved by them as it is by Christians.

Muslims

The Islamic faith is world-wide, and there are many adherents in Great Britain. It has rules on the practice of life which the faithful Muslim must follow, and the ones with which the nurse is most likely to come into contact relate to prayer and the diet.

The Muslim should pray five times a day at set times, preferably in a mosque. If this is not possible, he ought to use his prayer mat, washing himself, and facing towards Mecca; that is, in this country, towards the East. If he is unable through illness to do this, he may pray from his bed, again preferably with the foot of the bed towards Mecca.

The fast of Ramadan is required of all Muslims, who do not eat or drink in the daylight hours in the month of Ramadan. It is not obligatory for the sick to fast, though some Muslims in hospital may wish to do so. Muslims, like Jews, do not eat pork or bacon, and only eat meat from animals that have been bled.

The Imam is the Muslim priest, and the family may wish to have him present when death is imminent. Those around the bedside recite 'Kalana' aloud, and encourage the patient to do the same, so that he may die as a Muslim. It is usual for the relatives to wash the body ready for burial, wrap it in a shroud, and leave it with the feet pointing towards Mecca. Nurses should consult the family, and try to meet all of their wishes. Post-mortem examination is not allowed, nor the use of organs for transplant. Female Muslims must not after death be touched by male nurses, and vice versa.

Hindus

Hindus do not have an organised church, and their beliefs about the structure of society according to the caste system are not likely to be of relevance in hospital. They believe in an afterlife, which entails the transmigration of the soul. They are vegetarians, with an especial reverence for the cow, which is a holy animal.

The family should be consulted about their wishes for the patient. A Hindu priest may be called, who places water in the patient's mouth, and if he ties a thread around the wrist or neck, it is important not to remove it. The relatives may want to prepare the body and this should be allowed. Cremation is practised, and mourning lasts for ten days, after which the soul is believed to be back on the life cycle.

Buddhists

Buddhists seek to follow the founder of their religion in reaching enlightenment by keeping his precepts. They do not take life, so are vegetarians. There are no sacraments or special rites at death, but the body is usually prepared for cremation by the relatives. The thumbs and great toes are tied together with a hair from the head of one of the deceased's children. Death is usually accepted calmly and quietly.

Non-religious patients

There are large numbers of people who do not have any religious beliefs, and who do not expect any life when this one ends. Some call themselves atheists, and these are believers in a sense, since they actively believe that there is no God. Others speak of themselves as agnostics; they do not know; or as humanists, who want to benefit mankind. The ethical standards of behaviour of these people do not differ in any noticeable way from those who belong to a church and hope for eternal life. Like everyone else, they derive comfort from the loving presence of their family and friends, and the care of their nurses.

This brief account of religious beliefs refers to what nurses may find relevant in Great Britain, where the majority of people are at least nominally Christian. The trained nurse may find herself working in a Muslim country, or India, or Israel, and her standpoint and that of the community in which she is working will be on quite a different view of the norm.

2

The diagnosis of death

If we consult the dictionary for definitions of death, the results are unhelpful to nurses and doctors. Such definitions speak of the absence of life, cessation of living, and similar negative facts which do not provide criteria on which we can act. If someone has been dead for some hours, there is no doubt that life has ceased; the body heat has quite gone, breathing and pulse have stopped, rigor mortis has stiffened the joints. Someone who has been dead for longer than this will soon begin to show signs of decomposition in the colour of the skin. On the other hand, think of a patient on whom a heart operation on cardiopulmonary bypass has been performed. He is pulseless, cold, does not breathe, and there is no sign of brain activity in the electroencephalogram; all of which may indicate death in certain circumstances. No one in the theatre, however, is alarmed. When he is warmed, and taken off by-pass, his heart will resume beating. He will be connected to a ventilating machine until the next day, but then will resume breathing on his own.

The fear of being pronounced dead prematurely has long occupied men's minds, especially in the last century, when it was known for people to ask in their will that a vein be opened by a doctor before burial. Folk stories abound of Irishmen sitting up in their coffins in the middle of the funeral 'wake', and literature has many stories. It may be remembered how in *Ivanhoe* Athelstan regains consciousness while lying in state, because Sir Walter Scott could not bring himself to part with his Saxon hero.

Two factors have been responsible for the present continuing discussion on the diagnosis of death. The first is the ability by first aid and by more sophisticated methods to restore breathing and heartbeat to those in whom these functions have recently stopped, chiefly because of acute heart attacks, electric shock or other such emergencies. The second is the ability by life-support machines to maintain assisted respiration and heartbeat for quite long periods in those in whom they have ceased. As organ replacement surgery came into existence, and kidneys, cornea and even hearts might be taken from the recently dead under certain circumstances to aid the living, the problem became very acute and codes of practice to protect the very ill and their relatives were formulated.

Death usually occurs basically in one of three ways. The patient may die quite suddenly, sometimes with no previous symptoms. He may die from a fatal disease, like advanced cancer, and it is possible to note the signs of approaching death, and to forecast the likely time of death. Thirdly, he may be placed on a life-support machine following an accident or sudden emergency, and the criterion of brain death is now invoked to decide if death has occurred. This kind of event can only take place in hospital, probably in an intensive care unit.

Sudden death occurs not uncommonly; all nurses and many lay people have encountered it.

> A man lived a few miles from his elderly mother, and visited her quite frequently with his family, visits that gave her great pleasure. One day he and his wife and two children were going to have tea with her. When they rang the doorbell there was no answer, and on going round to the back they saw her in the lighted sitting room, in her chair beside the tea table. Her son broke a pane, opened the door, and they found her quite recently dead beside the meal she had prepared for them, with sandwiches, and cakes she had baked that morning.

This is probably the kind of departure most of us would like for ourselves, and although it is a shock for relatives at the time, it is well accepted later as a happy ending for the old or infirm. An increasing number of men in their thirties and forties suffer attacks of coronary thrombosis, and when help is at hand if they have cardiac arrest, the heart may be restarted, and the patient restored.

Many people have survived such incidents to live a normal life for years. These are the ones who have suffered cardiac standstill as a reaction to not very extensive disease, or as a result of electric shock or even drowning. Those who had (for instance) massive coronary occlusion or pulmonary thrombosis cannot be revived. It is also a prerequisite that resuscitation is begun very soon after cardiac arrest as the brain will not recover from a long period of anoxia.

When should efforts at resuscitation be given up? It is a doctor who decides that death has occurred, and in a developed country, medical help is soon available. If the arrest occurs in a ward, a doctor will be at hand immediately an emergency call is made. If it occurs somewhere else, an ambulance call will lead to a swift transfer to hospital. In general, if there is no heartbeat after five minutes, it is unlikely that recovery will result.

When cardiac resuscitation became widely known and accepted, nurses felt a lot of bewilderment about who should receive this treatment. A student nurse said to her teacher, 'People don't die now; they have cardiac arrest. Sometimes it's permanent'. While senior nurses and doctors hoped they would never be subjected to it, juniors sometimes felt rather confusedly that to deny it to anyone who collapsed suddenly was almost the equivalent of performing euthanasia.

With practice and knowledge, the circumstances in which it should not be applied have become clearer. It is inappropriate for anyone in the later stages of an incurable disease. If someone is approaching death in the manner described in the next section, to practise resuscitation if the heart stops unexpectedly, and to disturb the calm and peace of the last few hours by the commotion inevitably associated with this procedure, is unseemly and unnecessary.

The second way in which death comes is that which forms the major part of this book. It comes often at the end of an illness that may extend over years, and of which the end is foreseen. Sometimes it is the result of an infection for which treatment is unavailing. There is a period in which the management of distressing symptoms is the nurse's paramount concern, and the relations of the patient's family with the nursing and medical staff are very important, so that they understand what is happening.

As life fails, the pulse becomes weaker and faster. Respiration becomes shallow, involving only the upper part of the chest. The extremities and then the whole skin become cold, and sweating becomes marked as the body heat fails to evaporate it. Other movements cease, the half-open eyes are fixed. Consciousness is not always lost, and the patient may react to a word spoken to him at quite a late stage. The breathing becomes shorter and less frequent, and its cessation, sometimes after a last sighing, stertorous breath or the disappearance of the heartbeat marks the end of life. If the doctor is not present he will be summoned and pronounce life extinct.

Very often the relatives will be present when an expected death of this kind happens. They should be allowed some time alone, so that they can take in the fact that life is over, and also that they can see their relative in his natural state. The next morning, if they see him in the mortuary chapel, he will be laid out for burial in a formal way, already withdrawn from them.

The third way in which death occurs is the one in which most questions arise about diagnosis of whether life is extinct. It is the patient whose vital functions are maintained by machines, such as a respirator and a pacemaker. Such people have perhaps suffered injury (especially head injury) or cardiac operations, or acute heart attacks. Once respiration and circulation are being cared for and an intravenous line has been established, assessment of injuries, of signs of activity, and of the likely outcome can be made.

Three types of such outcome can be seen in patients having artificial ventilation. In the most favourable type consciousness is regained, and there is eventual recovery to normal health. In the second class recovery also occurs, but the patient is left with some brain damage. These are sad circumstances, and should make us resolve to do all we can to minimise the number of accidents (e.g. to motor-cyclists) which produce head injuries.

The third series is of people who do not respond to ventilation, and the dilemma of those caring for such people was severe. When did death occur? No one wants to add to the pain of relatives by continuing to ventilate a dead person, but neither doctors nor relatives want to give up if there is any hope that life is still present. Until firm criteria for the diagnosis of death were formulated, nurses had a feeling that switching off the life-support machines was the cause of death.

These anxieties and problems have existed ever since artificial ventilation began to be used, but the problem became more acute when transplant surgery became common. The supply of organs in good condition might give sight or life itself to the transplant surgeon's patients, but the duties of the doctors and nurses of the ventilated patient were to him and to his relatives and any suspicion of a hasty presumption of death, however unfounded, must be avoided. Turning off the switch must come after a firm diagnosis of death; it must be seen not as the cause of death, but as recognition that death has already occurred.

Brain Damage

The Royal Colleges which are the professional organisations of doctors held conferences on this subject and the British Code of Practice on the diagnosis of death was established in 1979. These criteria have been tested by continuing to ventilate those who have been deemed dead according to them, and in no case has the diagnosis been wrong.

The question of brain death arises under these circumstances:

1. If the patient is deeply unconscious and breathing is being maintained by a ventilator.

2. If a firm diagnosis has been made that the cause of the coma is irreversible brain damage.

These are the basic tests and observations which must be made and recorded in writing.

The investigations are undertaken by the physicians and surgeons caring for the patient, and they must have no connection with the transplant team. There are circumstances which render these tests invalid, and these circumstances must be excluded before the tests are administered:

1. The patient must not be suffering from hypothermia (i.e. have a low body temperature), which can help to produce suspended animation.

2. The patient must not be suffering from a drug overdose or intoxication. These are important exclusions; many people sustain injuries while intoxicated with alcohol or come in unconscious as the result of taking an drug overdose.

3. No drug should have been administered within the last eight hours; this is especially important with regard to muscle relaxants.

When these circumstances have been excluded, the relatives are told that the doctors feel that the patient is in fact dead, and that tests are going to be made to ascertain if that is so. These tests will be repeated later in order to make sure that no change has taken place. Two doctors undertake the tests and one must have been qualified for at least five years. Six facts must be established if death is to be presumed:

1. There is no spontaneous respiration when the ventilator is disconnected. The normal stimulus to respiration is the level of carbon dioxide in the blood. The way of ensuring this is to ventilate the patient with 100% oxygen for 10 minutes and then on 5% carbon dioxide with oxygen for five minutes. The ventilator is disconnected and the patient observed for signs of spontaneous breathing. If none occur ventilation is resumed and the rest of the tests carried out.

2. The pupils are dilated and fixed; there is no pupillary reaction to light.

3. The conjunctival reflex is absent; there is no lid reaction when each cornea is touched.

4. The vestibulo-ocular response is absent. A syringe of ice-cold water is injected into each ear and produces no eye movement.

5. Pain reflexes are absent, e.g. there is no head movement in response to pressure over the supraorbital nerve.

6. The gag reflex is absent; there is no response to bronchial stimulation by a suction catheter.

Ventilation is continued while the relatives are told the result. The relatives should be in privacy, and sitting down when they are informed as sympathetically as possible by one of the doctors that their tests indicate that the patient is dead, but that the tests will be repeated later. At this time the question of the use of organs for transplant can be raised and is indeed sometimes raised by the relatives themselves. It is not advisable to ask about this while the patient is 'alive', it may give the impression that surgeons have an interest in his death. There will be time to inform the transplant team that organs may shortly be available. After the tests have been repeated and death confirmed, the ventilator can be switched off when the transplant team is ready to remove the organs.

This is a time of great stress for the relatives. The accident itself has come as a shock, the news that it may prove fatal, and finally that the patient is dead, are other severe blows. Sometimes they ask the doctor if he is quite sure, and he can stress that the tests are to be repeated later. It must be fully explained that the movement of the chest induced by the respirator is not really breathing and that switching off is not the termination of the patient's life; that has already happened.

Whether the relatives are present or not depends on their wishes. Some may wish to be there, and wish the priest to be present. Many are deeply relieved by the silence that ensues when the respirator stops. Others do not wish to be present, and in this case the apparatus should be cleared away, and the patient left looking as peaceful as possible before they come in for a farewell.

It will be seen that there is no reference to the electroencephalogram (e.e.g.) in the criteria of death, though of course an e.e.g. is frequently used in investigtion of unconscious people. Occasional flickers may be seen on an e.e.g.; it is the concept of death of the brain stem which involves all the vital functions, that is held to be crucial in this country. In others (e.g. in Eastern Europe) e.e.g. is deemed necessary.

It is a great comfort to the family to see the patient receiving nursing care right to the end. The death of a patient for whom the medical team may have worked very hard is disheartening. Superintendents of intensive care units must be alert to the needs of nurses as well as of patients and relatives. They must see that nurses fully understand the concept of brain death and do not feel there is any element of ending the patient's life when the ventilator is disconnected.

3

Stillbirth and cot death

Babies may die before birth, or in infancy, sometimes from causes that are imperfectly understood. The parents, grand-parents and other children will have need of understanding and support. Nurses, midwives and health visitors should study the problems involved and the common reactions, and be prepared to help with them. People who have lost a baby often complain of the lack of information and communication from their professional attendants. It is understandable that neighbours and friends should feel diffident about raising the topic of a lost baby, but nurses should be able to approach bereaved parents without embarrassment, and offer genuine understanding.

Stillbirth

Stillbirth is not uncommon; about six thousand babies die before or at birth every year in this country, so midwives may expect to encounter this. Sometimes it is known that the baby has died before labour begins, and it is inevitable that labour and delivery will be rather melancholy. A bonus point is that the choice of analgesic does not depend on the wellbeing of the baby and the mother can be kept well sedated. It is to be hoped that the father can be present to share the experience with his wife, as he will then understand it better. The hoped-for cry of the newly delivered baby will not occur, but it is desirable not to conduct the delivery in silence, and gentle, quiet and reassuring comment and instruction given.

If the baby dies during delivery the situation is more tense and more emotional. Monitoring techniques will usually indicate that there is fetal distress, and the mother soon begins to pick up the signs of anxiety among the delivery team. If the baby is born naturally, she asks 'Is the baby all right?' as she does not hear the expected cry. She should be told that the doctors and midwives are working on the baby's problems. This especially applies if there are congenital deformities, which may be incompatible with life, or may be of a kind that will be distressing but not life-threatening, for instance a cleft lip.

As stillbirth is not infrequent, staff should have a policy on how to fill the bereaved parents' needs, based on knowledge of these. The mother should be told as soon as possible; if the father was present at the birth, and both can be told together, this is helpful. There is no doubt that staff feel that a stillbirth is a kind of defeat, and are apt to be rather defensive about what may be seen as a professional failure. No hint of this feeling should be shown to the parents, and we must not be afraid to show warmth and sympathy. When the mother's toilet has been completed she should, if possible, be taken to a single room, made comfortable in bed, and left alone with her husband. To send her back to a ward of mothers and babies is cruel.

The first response by the parents, especially the mother, is a state of shock. They feel cold, sick and confused, sighing and perhaps weeping. The nurse may offer both a hot drink and assure them that she is near at hand if wanted, and then leave them for ten minutes or so. The father should not be sent away until he wants to go; when it is necessary to give nursing care to the mother, he may be reminded that perhaps there are people to whom he should telephone. Consideration should always be given about the parents' seeing the dead baby. It is a subject to which parents often refer in later years. They should be asked what they would like to do, and nurses should encourage them to believe that whichever they do is right, and should not press their own views. If a baby is deformed, it may not seem desirable to the nurse for the mother to see it, but it is possible by judicious arrangement of sheets and pads to allow a partial view of even a severely abnormal child. The important thing is that the parents choose what to do, and are then supported in the decision as the right one for them.

The physical care that the mother is given will follow the usual obstetric principles. Observation is made to ensure that the uterus is well contracted, that the bladder is emptied within a few hours of delivery, and toilet of the perineum is performed. Milk will be secreted by the breasts, and the mother often finds it distressing that her body behaves as if the baby were alive. Lactation suppressants may be ordered, a supporting brassiere worn, and she is advised not to express milk even if the breasts are tense, as this will prolong secretion. The diminution of the lochia, and the involution of the uterus are noted by the visiting midwife, and the usual postnatal visit to the obstetrician after six weeks is booked. This visit is a very important one; not only is the physical condition checked, but time allowed for discussion to find how the parents are adjusting. The question of a further pregnancy can be raised, and if the stillbirth was due to a deformity, genetic counselling can be offered.

The father's role at this time is a difficult one. He must support and comfort his wife, and also undertake practical and painful duties. For instance, the baby's birth must be registered as a stillbirth. The doctor gives the husband a certificate, which must be taken to the Registrar of Births, Marriages and Deaths. If the baby was alive when born, but died immediately afterwards, the doctor supplies a death certificate and the Registrar will then give a certificate for burial.

The arrangements for burial should be discussed with the hospital secretary or administrator. The hospital can, if the parents wish, arrange for burial or cremation without charge. Some parents may wish to have a burial service and to know where the baby is buried, and in this case the certificate is given to an undertaker, who makes the arrangements. Some parents wish to give the baby a name, especially if they have discussed names during pregnancy.

It will usually be the father's task to tell the grandparents, and perhaps also other children in the family. Close friends must also be told, and perhaps a decision made· about arrangements at home for the new arrival who will not now be returning, by way of baby clothes or furnishings.

Psychological reactions

Immediately after the first shock is over, parents ask 'Why did it happen?' or 'Why did it happen to us?' and they seek for causes in themselves or in the medical or nursing staff. The opportunity for full and frank discussion may prevent long term problems of adjustment. If the child had a deformity which was not compatible with life, the stillbirth may be easier to understand, but raises many other questions.

The two commonest feelings in the early stage are guilt and anger, and in the interests of a successful long-term adjustment, both must be understood and dealt with. Couples who have had intercourse in the later days of pregnancy often feel this must be the cause, and must be assured that this is irrelevant. Sometimes the mother has made half-hearted efforts to induce a period in the early days of conception with aperients or hot baths. This too is irrelevant. The history of the pregnancy is searched for possible causes; did she take too much exercise or too little, or smoke a cigarette, or go swimming? It is better to discuss such points fully or they will become fixed in irrational beliefs that may cause pain for years.

Anger is often directed against the doctors and midwives, who are accused of some failure of attention or method. The nurse must understand this feeling, and not let it arouse anger in herself, but should answer that she is sorry they feel this way, and that she can understand why they do, though she does not accept the accusations.

Grief over the loss of a baby is natural, and a period of mourning must be endured. Mothers often think of the baby for years, and imagine how he may have grown and developed. Fathers too may have fantasies about the child, and imagine taking a boy around and teaching him sports. Such ideas are not harmful if they do not dominate the mind or spoil the relation with other children.

If the parents already have children who are old enough to know that a little brother or sister was going to arrive, they will be confused and unhappy. Young children are often jealous at the thought of a risk of mother's love being transferred to a new baby, and after a stillbirth may fear that their thoughts have led to the death of the sibling.

It will be seen that many people are involved in the emotion engendered by a stillbirth. Friends are apt to say to the bereaved parents, 'You are young, you will have another baby'. This may be true, but it should never be suggested that this one will replace the lost one. It will be loved for its own sake. Once the normal period of grieving is over, the memory will take a normal place in the past, if the problems associated with it have been thoughtfully and sensitively handled at the time of the stillbirth.

Cot Death

This term describes a tragic event that occurs once in about every five hundred births in this country. It is known all over the world, and in every class of society. The typical story is that a baby of between a month and a year old, apparently perfectly healthy, is put to sleep in its cot after a feed, and a few hours later is found to be dead. Post-mortem examination sometimes reveals inflammation in the lungs or the meninges, but it may be so slight that it is difficult to feel that it is the direct cause of death. Some feel that there has been a respiratory or cardiac arrest, such as sometimes occurs in adults after trivial operations.

Since the cause of cot deaths is not known, it is not possible to do anything specific to prevent it, and the nurse's responsibility is the care of the parents, and any others who may have been concerned. Apart from the grief involved, guilt is obviously going to be experienced. Could the death have been avoided if the mother had looked at the baby more often? If the baby was in the temporary care of grandparents or a baby sitter, was the mother at fault in leaving the baby to others?

A woman who has a stillbirth feels that the baby she carried was part of herself for a long time, but she can only speculate on how he would have developed. A baby who dies in its cot has a name, and a personality and ways of his own, and the loss is all the more poignant.

An inquest is always held, and the coroner does his best to see that the parents are not made to feel in any way to blame. Some have a leaflet to give to a bereaved couple, and it may be a comfort to realise that cot death is a recognised medical entity. Some may like to be put in touch with the Foundation for the Study of Infant Deaths, 5th floor, 4 Grosvenor Place, London SW1 7HD. Health visitors, doctors and ministers of religion may be able to offer comfort. Mourning, it must be remembered, is normal and cannot be hastened.

If there are other children in the family, they must be given loving comfort. Young ones may feel that they too are threatened with sudden death, and older ones who felt sibling jealousy of the new baby may feel that somehow they caused the death.

The question of having another baby must be faced eventually. It must never be suggested that another baby could fill the place of the one who died, but if the couple wanted a child, they will still want one. It is difficult not to feel acute anxiety, or to watch over the new baby, and wake to look at him in the night. Baby-monitoring equipment is sometimes loaned by maternity hospitals to mothers who have experienced a cot death. Some women find this relieves to some extent their fears that they are not taking every possible precaution, while others find that listening for the alarm increases their anxiety. The system is liable to false alarms, like the cardiac monitoring equipment in an intensive care unit, and this can be very frightening.

If possible, the new baby should sleep in a different room, or in a cot in a different position, so that the chain of painful memories is interrupted. The health visitor should visit regularly, and assess the mother's need for support and reassurance.

Appropriate Treatment

In several places in this book, allusion is made to the time when a decision has to be taken as to whether it is realistic or helpful to continue active treatment of a disease, when the patient who is suffering from the disease is obviously soon going to die because of it. Sometimes this decision has to be made not towards the end of an illness, but at the very beginning of life.

Babies are sometimes born with deformities which can be recognised at birth. These may be so severe that they are incompatible with life outside the uterus, and the baby dies immediately after birth. Some are comparatively trivial — an extra finger, for instance. Some, like hare lip and cleft palate, are disfiguring but can be corrected by surgery later. There are some, however, in which there is a congenital abnormality which must result in severe handicap.

An instance of such handicap might be spina bifida, with a lumbar meningomyelocele. The spinal nerves are involved in this condition, and it may be obvious at birth that there is paraplegia, and that the baby will not walk, or be continent.

Such severely handicapped babies are commonly born in a state of shock, and do not breathe spontaneously. Is it appropriate treatment to revive the baby and seek to start respiration? Once the first steps have been taken it is difficult not to continue technical treatment.

Obstetricians and neonatal paediatricians should have a policy about what measures should be taken to revive and keep alive handicapped babies who cannot perform their basic functions. The official guidelines issued some years ago advise that doctors do not use unusual technical care in prolonging life for the grossly deformed, and most doctors would appear to agree. Nurses should understand and accept the views of their colleagues, but should be free to ask questions and express their feelings and to seek more like-minded colleagues if necessary.

It must be recognised that not all doctors and nurses would agree with the *laissez-faire* attitude and would not adopt it. They would not think that ventilation or intubation were extraordinary measures, and would defend their views ably.

Some deformities can be recognised before birth, by amniocentesis, and the parents can be offered the option of termination of pregnancy. Not all mothers have amniocentesis, and not all of these would accept abortion, and the problems of severe congenital handicap will be with us for a long time.

The easiest cases are those in which the baby shows no sign of life at birth. The parents have the same sense of loss and grief as others who have had a still birth, perhaps lessened somewhat by the realisation that the baby has been saved suffering. They will however ask questions about how the deformity was caused, whether it was somehow their fault, and they will be in need of guidance as to how to think and feel, and to prevent guilt. They will also need genetic counselling about the risks attached to future pregnancies.

The topic of the survival prospects of severely deformed children has received much attention in literature and on television. The amount of technical information and ability to diagnose and treat increases all the time, and raises problems that previously were hardly thought of. Parents, doctors and nurses must exchange information and thoughts, and perhaps recognise that there are honestly held views that cannot be reconciled. Some may feel that life must be preserved if it can be; others that the costs may be too high. We must remember that neither side has a monopoly of concern and loving kindness.

The ventilation in the press and even in the law courts of the problems of the severely handicapped neonate and his family, and how medical and nursing staff should reach decisions about these, may produce conflicting and emotional expressions of opinion. Such public discussion has the important function of bringing information on the thoughts and feelings of ordinary lay people to the notice of professionals. Those who work in obstetric and baby units may encounter these problems quite frequently, while workers in other fields may never meet them at all. All of us should however read the nursing and lay papers and discuss with colleagues, so that our professional and social policies are soundly and ethically based.

Nurses who are in any doubt about their position with regard to medical directions or practices should consult their nursing officer. The Hospital Ethical Committee may have a useful part to play in helping staff to formulate practice which is humane and ethical. Nurses might need information in some circumstances about their legal responsibilities, and this can be supplied by their professional organisation.

4

Care in terminal illness

Birth and death are often spoken about as natural events that mark our entry into this life and our departure from it. Up to this century, both were domestic happenings; most people died at home. The expectation of life for men in 1900 was 48 years; it has risen now to 68 years, chiefly because the acute infections that killed young people have been conquered. While a number of people die suddenly in accidents or from heart attacks, most people in this country will live into old age, and probably many of them will spend their last days in hospital or a hospice, and it is the principles of nursing care for these which will be discussed here.

The number of hospices has increased because it is felt that the busy, acute hospital, geared to resuscitation and life-support systems, is less able to provide the atmosphere and multiple skills involved than a hospice specialising in such care.

Effective terminal care involves not only looking after someone in his last illness, but also helping his family in the short-term conditions of bereavement and in their continuing problems. The difficulties of staff in situations of terminal care must also be considered if such care is to be effective, and by 'staff' is implied not only nurses, but doctors, social workers, chaplains, and domestic staff.

The skills and abilities required of the nurse can be summarised as follows:

For the patient

1. To make a plan of nursing care based on a nursing history and observations of the physical and psychological symptoms shown.

2. To discuss with the doctors the extent of the patient's knowledge of his state in order to ensure truthful relations. To cooperate with the medical staff in a drug regime and other methods which will effectively control pain and other distressing symptoms. This is central to compassionate care.

3. To acquire skills in conversing with the dying which will enable the patient to ask questions and express fears, and to have these questions directed to doctor, chaplain or social worker if necessary.

4. To be able to complete the last offices after death for people of any or no religion in accordance with their beliefs.

5. To be aware of the legal and ethical problems that may arise in connection with such problems as making wills, or requests for euthanasia.

In no other branch of nursing is it more important to make a detailed plan based on the patient's needs. We can probably agree that he would hope for freedom from disturbing symptoms, especially pain and sleeplessness, and peace of mind for himself and his relatives.

'Terminal' care implies that active attempts at cure have ceased, and a patient admitted for such care must be told the truth about his condition if he asks for it. No attempt should be made to force a diagnosis on someone who does not wish to discuss it, but deception will destroy the basis of trust between patient and his attendants. It must not be thought that knowing that he has incurable cancer means that he will accept the fact with resignation; some respond with anger and bitterness, blaming other hospitals, or God. Such reactions must be accepted with understanding and compassion. From the initial interview, from the family, or by observation, as full a picture as possible is built up, so that a detailed care plan is devised. We shall want to know if pain is prominent, and where it is situated; whether secondary growths are present and their situation; if there is fluid in the peritoneal or pleural cavities; if there are stomata or drainage tubes; if he suffers from breathlessness, nausea, vomiting, constipation, incontinence; what is the state of his nutrition, and of the skin of his pressure areas; does he sleep well, and has he an appetite; is there any loss of sight or hearing that might make communication difficult; does he get up at all, or is he bedfast. His religion will have been noted, and if he has one it may play an important part in his adjustment.

All dying patients need the opportunity to express themselves, and plenty of time should be given to listening. Chaplains of all denominations are regular visitors, skilled listeners, and able to provide spiritual comfort. Doctors must often spend a long time on talk with their patients and nurses who are constantly with their patients must expect to play a major role in listening. Young nurses often feel inadequate at the thought of counselling the dying, but must remember that listening and encouraging the patient to express his thoughts is far more important than offering their own opinions.

For the relatives

1. To understand the common reaction to impendng bereavement, and to offer sympathy and help.
2. To know the agencies and people which may be of longer-term assistance.

Once the patient is free from pain, his family have a great fear removed but they have to face the fact that bereavement is inevitable. They are given every opportunity to visit, and their comfort is considered in all ways. Relatives sometimes seem critical and hostile to staff, but this is due either to grief, or to subconscious feelings of guilt that they are unable to care for the patient themselves. An opportunity to help in giving meals, or with washing, may be welcome and provide them with a role.

Nurses in a ward usually do not see the relatives again once the patient has died, but their need is at its greatest in the ensuing weeks or months. A hospice social worker may visit, and the health visitor may be informed if further support is necessary. Old people who have lost a lifelong partner may be introduced to a social group or given information about Cruse, an organisation to help bereaved women.

For the staff

To recognise that staff also suffer from grief, and to look out for signs of strain in all grades of colleague, and to know how to offer support.

In most branches of medicine, nurses and doctors are encouraged by hopes of curing people, but this reward is not present here. By definition, those needing terminal care will all die quite soon, and the aim must be that the patient departs in peace, unmarred by pain or any physical troubles we can alleviate, and that the family share in the peace and are helped to face bereavement and grief. It would however be unusual for someone to spend long in this work without feelings of depression and strain from time to time. All members of staff should support each other at such times, above all listening with sympathy. The feelings of domestic staff are often similar to those of the nurses, as they often form bonds of sympathy with patients and their families, and the ward sister must watch them in case they need support.

Evaluation of the success of the nursing plan for the terminally ill should always be undertaken at ward meetings. It cannot be hoped that success will invariably be achieved, however devoted the care given, and the reasons for failure to achieve the aim for the patient or his relatives should be sought, in the hope of avoiding them in the future.

Giving Physical Care

The principles of planning and giving nursing care to a patient who is going to die resemble in many respects those which apply to nursing people who have an acute illness, or one which will not shorten their life. We aim to prevent discomforts or pain arising, or to treat them if they do, but there is very rarely any need to proffer care that the patient who is dying dislikes or fears. Sometimes it is necessary when caring for someone in an acute illness, or following an operation, to urge activity that is in the patient's long term interests, but against his inclination. He is asked to stand out of bed or walk, even if he has an intravenous infusion or must take a bladder drainage bag with him, in order to avoid deep venous thrombosis. Uncomfortable investigations may have to be performed, because they may yield information that will lead to diagnosis and eventual cure. Powerful drugs may have disagreeable side-effects that the patient must be encouraged to endure. This is not the case with the dying patient; the nursing care is all comfort-giving, and centred on the wishes of the patient himself. Everything that is done should be for his peace and well-being.

In some ways decisions are simplified; for instance, there is no need to ask oneself if resuscitation should be attempted if the patient should suddenly cease to breathe. On the other hand, there is never a time when physical care is not required, or the nurse says, 'There is nothing more I can do'. Each part of the body contributes to the wellbeing of the whole. Failure to treat an infected mouth may lead to dehydration and its attendant wretchedness. A loaded rectum has far-reaching effects, mental and physical. Patient-centred activity in no way implies inactivity, but the direction of our skills to supplying the wants we can recognise, even if the patient does not.

It is sometimes felt that nursing the dying implies an emphasis on spiritual rather than physical care; this is not true. Both aspects are interdependent. The person who is not disturbed by pain, discomfort or physical indignity is able, if he wishes, to give thought to other matters, and with more effect. The last weeks and days have to be *lived*, and in many cases can be a time of peace, and of happiness in the love of friends and family, if we are able to give physical ease. The old Anglican evening prayer asks that it may be granted to us 'to pass our time in rest and quietness', and this is what we aim to give our patient by our expert care.

Activity

This is an area in which the wishes of the patient are the primary consideration. Some people feel a desire to remain active, and not to be totally bedfast until it cannot be avoided. We might remember Emily Bronte, who got up and dressed on the day of her death, and only consented to go to bed in the last hour of her life.

If the possibility of short outings is actively considered and a little imagination used, much happiness can be given. Short outings in a wheelchair to the garden or grounds, to enjoy fresh air and a change of surroundings along with the family, can be a source of great pleasure. Outings by car, a few hours at home, or even a visit to a play or concert may be possible. People sometimes feel when they begin their last illness 'I am going to be here until I die', and to find, when their pain and symptoms are adequately controlled, that a change of scene is still possible can give a great lift to the spirits.

Getting up is perhaps easier at home, where the surroundings are familiar and beloved, rather than in a hospital ward, where the alternative to staying in bed is to sit in a chair beside the bed. If a patient wishes to sit up, a comfortable chair and sufficient covers should be provided, and if relatives are present, a little area can perhaps be devised where the group can be together in close proximity. People in terminal heart failure are often more comfortable sitting up in a chair than in bed, and may spend most of their time sitting up. A cantilever table in front of them on which they can lean and support the shoulder girdle is an added comfort.

Those who do not wish to get up need not be urged to do so. They may want to pass their time resting.

Skin Care

Nurses tend to feel that those who are confined to bed require a daily bed bath. Many patients feel the same; they have been used to a bath or shower every day, and would feel a lack if this were denied to them. To some, however, it is a tedious chore, disturbing not relaxing, and consuming strength they can ill afford and, to these, bed baths may be given less frequently. Local washing daily after bowel action is desirable, and refreshing of the face and hands is always welcome.

Nurses may also like to consider whether the patient's view that washing is tiresome is not a comment on the nurse's technique, and that plenty of hot water, deftness, minimum exposure, and less demands on movement by the patient would not modify his opinion. Everyone likes putting the hands in water, and the feet too can be immersed without much difficulty. There are hoists for putting the helpless into the bath if it seems for their benefit, and baths into which patients can be put on a stretcher are available in specialist institutions.

Giving a bed bath provides an opportunity for inspecting sacrum, heels, trochanters and elbows for signs of irritation by pressure, and if a bath is not given daily, this should be done while making the bed. Finger nails may become grimy even when there is no physical activity, and should be looked at daily, and cleaned with a moistened orange stick.

If the skin is generally dry, baby oil can be added to the washing water. Arachis oil can be massaged into dry areas, and women may like one of the many moisturising body lotions available.

Clean nails, fresh bedclothes and well groomed hair provide a ready guide to the standard of care a helpless person is receiving. Men should be shaved regularly. Women's hair is brushed into the style to which they are accustomed, if possible. If a patient wants a shampoo it can usually be given, and if it is felt that the hair of a patient in terminal care needs freshening, the comb can be moistened in surgical spirit, or eau de Cologne. People who have cancer may have had cytotoxic drugs that caused the hair to fall out. Men usually seem not to care too much about this, but women usually want to have their heads covered. They may not want to be bothered with a wig at this stage, but a pretty scarf, or boudoir or shower cap may be acceptable as an alternative. Those who like perfume should continue to use it.

Mouth Care

This is a very important element in the nursing plan. There are many factors that may lead to a dry, unpleasant, uncomfortable mouth. Lack of appetite, lowered fluid intake, and mouth breathing in the later stages may contribute to it. Candidiasis (thrush) is not uncommon in dying patients, especially if they have been receiving cytotoxic drugs or broad spectrum antibiotics. The diagnosis is easily made by observing white patches on the tongue and inside of the cheeks, and regular observation with a pencil torch and spatula should be made in order to detect it early. The current treatment for thrush is given two hourly; a mouth wash, such as Oraldene or Compound Thymol Glycerin, is given first and this is followed by Nystatin (100 000 units in 1 ml) which is given undiluted, swilled round the mouth and swallowed. If the infection does not respond to this fungicide, miconazole (Daktarin Gel) 5 ml is used two or four hourly.

Dentures should be worn unless the patient chooses otherwise. They improve the appearance, assist in eating, and raise the morale. If mouth breathing causes dryness, glycerine or soft paraffin can be applied to the lips. The nurse has a variety of methods of dealing with a dry mouth. Pieces of ice flavoured with lemon or orange juice are refreshing to suck. Those with their own teeth may like to have them brushed with dentifrice if they are unable to do it for themselves, and an electric toothbruth is effective and easy to use.

Food and Drink

This term is used rather than the more austere 'diet', which is only required for a minority of people in their final illness. Diabetics need their diet, and if the patient has renal, or hepatic failure, some dietetic control may be necessary to avoid the occurrence of fits. Small quantities of appetising, easily digested foods should be given as long as the patient wants them. Relatives often like to bring small items they know he is fond of, and giving food expresses their need to offer some service. Slices of peeled orange, seedless grapes and peeled peach segments are often acceptable if given in very small quantities, whereas bowls of fruit may stay uneaten on the locker.

The fluids given offer opportunity for imagination by staff and relations. Oranges can be pressed to provide fresh juice, and milk shakes, icy cold, are often liked. Many people retain an appreciation of smell, and aromatic soups or fresh coffee may be taken with pleasure. Those who have been used to alcohol will appreciate a little, and 15 or 30 ml of brandy is a good sedative for the elderly at night.

Bowel Regulation

Failure to understand the necessity for bowel action by the terminally ill is an important cause of misery and indignity. It is often believed that the faeces represent food residue only, and that someone who is not taking normal quantities of food will have nothing to eliminate. This is far from the truth;

bacteria, epithelial cells and mucus form an important part of the stool, and unless evacuated will accumulate in hardening masses in the rectum, and extend from there into the pelvic colon and even further unless the condition is treated.

The results of neglect to maintain normal bowel action may have far-reaching effects. Colonic pain and nausea will remove the appetite, and dehydration will harden still further the impacted faeces. Incontinence of urine is often caused by pressure of the loaded rectum on the bladder base. Faecal-stained fluid escapes from the dilated anal sphincter, and is labelled faecal incontinence. It may lead to soreness of the skin, and even breakdown of the skin. Mental confusion is seen in severe cases.

Staff in hospices are well aware of the importance to the general well-being of maintaining evacuation, and are often disturbed by the number of patients who reach them from home and even hospital with impacted faeces. Once the stage of overflow faecal incontinence is reached, people find it difficult to realise that their patient needs aperients, or enemata, or even manual evacuation of the rectum. Records may show that the patient has had several fluid 'stools' a day, but such statements are meaningless as an account of the normal physiology of the colon.

The selection of an aperient requires great care. Liquid paraffin or Milpar is inadequate, and by leaking past the solid material in the rectum may make matters even more difficult. Stool softeners like Dorbanex Forte or Dioctyl Forte are useful, and may have to be used regularly, especially if the patient is having opiates for the relief of pain, as so many of them do. Regular assessment of the colonic function makes an essential contribution to the patient's comfort, and avoids painful and undignified side-effects.

Incontinence

Incontinence of urine causes distress and feelings of humiliation in those who experience it. The cause must be ascertained by taking a history, and by noting when it occurs. It has already been said that faecal impaction is a common cause in the terminally ill if colonic function has not been well managed, and this should be one of the first points to be investigated.

The emotional state may allow incontinence; people who are wretched or apathetic on account of mental problems or physical ones may regress to an infantile state in which they urinate automatically. While it is not possible to bring peace of mind to all dying people, it is an aim we should keep before us. A bedpan or the use of a commode should be offered regularly.

The drugs given to relieve pain should not, if a good schedule has been devised, lead to stupor, but freedom from pain is more important than urinary continence.

An indwelling urethral catheter does not cause the discomforts once associated with this procedure. Silastic catheters are not irritating to mucous membranes, and can be retained without change for some weeks. This means that for most whose last illness may be associated in its closing phases with incontinence, one catheterisation is enough to keep them dry without discomfort. Daily cleaning of the catheter must be done. Some men find a condom with an attached drainage tube more acceptable than a catheter.

If catheterisation is not thought desirable, there are many commercial pads and dressings that allow urine to pass through, so that the skin does not become macerated. Nurses will not want to let the patient feel that his infirmity is a reproach in any way, and will care for him with tactful courtesy.

Faccal incontinence is less common, except an overflow from a loaded colon, which must be relieved. It may appear as a terminal symptom and, in these circumstances, sheets must be changed as soon as possible to avoid distress to relatives and maintain a good environment.

Prevention of Pressure Sores

Intelligent, insightful care must be given to promoting this aim. While there are many areas from which skin can be lost in special circumstances, the skin over the sacrum, great trochanters and heels is the most vulnerable. Most patients who are dying will have a low score on the Norton Pressure Sore Assessment Scale (Table 1), and may well have additional handicaps, e.g. widespread malignant disease and emaciation.

Table 1   Norton pressure sore assessment scale

Physical condition		Mental condition		Activity		Mobility		Incontinent	
Good	4	Alert	4	Ambulant	4	Full	4	Not	4
Fair	3	Apathetic	3	Walk/help	3	Slightly limited	3	Occasionally	3
Poor	2	Confused	2	Chairbound	2	Very limited	2	Usually	2
Very bad	1	Stuporose	1	Bedfast	1	Immobile	1	Doubly	1

In using this scale the authors would like to acknowledge the work of Doreen Norton FRCN in this field. (Norton, D. (1975) Research and the problem of pressure sores. *Nursing Mirror*, **140(7)** Feb 13, pp 65–67.)

Relief of pressure by regular turning is the most important element of preventive action, and will normally be done two-hourly. Incontinence of urine and/or faeces may be successfully controlled, and will remove one hazard to the skin. Bedclothes can be supported by cradles. Fleeces, pads, sorbo rings and similar appliances are valuable and the use of a large-cell ripple mattress or a water bed is a great help. The skin must be kept clean, and powder will help to avoid friction. The use of spirit or soap, except for routine cleaning is usually too drying to be useful.

Sometimes a patient is admitted to a unit with pressure sores. The same principles of regular turning and the use of soft materials must be followed but, in addition, dressings to cure infection and to minimise pain are needed. Most experienced nurses have their favourite ways of dressing pressure sores, but it seems that it is the enthusiasm and devotion of the user that is more important than the medicament chosen.

Even if it is thought that someone has not long to live, pressure sores should be treated. The pain from these, and the results of infection, add to the patient's problems and to those of the nurse who is trying to solve them for him.

Relief of Pain

Pain is a common and very complex symptom, and its relief in the dying is one of the most important duties of doctors and nurses. While administration of an analgesic is a major consideration, it is by no means the only one, and sympathetic assessment of the cause and nature of the patient's reaction to his situation is required. Those who favour euthanasia usually speak of the right to be spared intolerable pain. People do indeed have the right to such relief, and it can be supplied by insightful, sympathetic and skillful management (p. 37).

There are three main components to severe pain:

1. That of the cause, which must be identified and if possible removed. This cannot be done for most pain associated with terminal illness, but is possible in quite a few ways. Some of the commoner types of pain are considered below.

2. Autonomic nervous system symptoms. Sweating, vomiting, tachycardia and fainting are well known examples. These symptoms are very distressing, and must be relieved.

3. Emotional reactions. The way in which a patient reacts to pain is not entirely due to its severity, were it possible to grade it, but also due to his feelings about it. Anxiety and fear are universally experienced by those in severe pain. Will the staff be able to relieve it? Will they give him medicine whenever he needs it? Does it mean that he is going to die soon? All of us know the pain in the chest ('heartache') that comes with grief, and separation from loved ones and fear of impending loss are felt by nearly all the terminally ill. While there are drugs that will alleviate depression and anxiety, full and free communication between patient and staff may allow some of these fears to be allayed. For instance, the patient may truthfully be assured that his pain will not merely be controlled, but prevented. Nurses often feel some anxiety themselves about how they are to deal with questions by the dying, but on the whole listening is much more important than learning clever techniques about answering, and by listening one often gains information that will help in giving effective assistance. Families too ask about pain, and can be given the same assurance that it can be prevented.

These are some of the types of pain which can occur in dying people as well as in others.

1. *Colic* or pain due to spasm and violent peristalsis in plain muscle. Colic due to intestinal obstruction by malignant involvement of the gut is an example of pain of which the cause cannot be removed. If the obstruction is low down, abdominal distention can be severe, and puncture of gas-

filled loops with a needle may be helpful. Colic due to severe constipation can of course be removed by treatment of the cause.

2. *Ischaemic pain*. If an organ or muscle is deprived of blood, intense pain is produced. The best known example is that caused by myocardial infarction, in which the pain is made worse by the feeling that the heart has been attacked, and that death may follow. Angina pectoris and leg cramp may occur in the dying, and should be treated by the appropriate drugs.

3. *Pain in bones*. This is commonly due to secondary deposits of malignant tissues, or to pathological fractures. Radiotherapy is quite effective in relieving the pain of new growth in bone, and if it is available may be ordered for this purpose, and not in hope of effecting a cure.

4. *Nerve pain*. This type can be very severe and intractable. Patients often speak of it as 'excruciating'. The pain of herpes zoster and trigeminal neuralgia are examples. In advanced malignant disease the roots of the spinal nerves may be involved, or plexuses (such as the brachial) or individual nerves like the sciatic. Interruption of the sensory pathway by which the pain reaches the brain may sometimes be successful. Nerve blocks and percutaneous cordotomy are examples of such action.

5. *Pain from trauma* is seen after surgical operations; wounds that are subject to movement from breathing, or to stretching by abdominal distention are painful. Some of the most painful traumatic conditions are those in which superficial injuries expose nerve endings, as in burns. Superficial skin loss over pressure areas is exceedingly painful, and every effort is made to spare the dying patient this extra burden.

Relief of pain in the incurably ill will require the use of analgesics, but there are many elements in distress, and these will vary from person to person. Breathlessness, nausea, sleeplessness and fear may all contribute to the patient's 'pain', and each symptom must be considered and dealt with. Simple medical measures like tapping an abdomen distended by ascites may greatly increase comfort. Nursing care in connection with posture in bed, mouth hygiene, and relief of pressure may make a significant contribution, and measures like heat, massage, and sympathetic encouragement should not be forgotten.

Analgesics

The drugs that relieve pain range from the simple and mild, such as aspirin, to the powerful opiates like morphine and diamorphine. In addition, there are drugs that can increase the sense of wellbeing and relieve symptoms, and thus reduce discomforts. Many analgesics are better for one purpose than another, and all have unwanted side-effects as well as the desired ones. The choice of the drug to be used; the dose, the interval and the route of administration are elements of the doctor's skill in prescribing. The observations of the nurses about the patient's reactions give him the information that is needed for a successful result.

The process is not a simple one of giving a chosen drug and increasing the dose as necessary. Indeed, once the patient has confidence that he is going to be relieved of pain, he may require less analgesic, not more. One person may value the drowsiness induced by the opiates, another may wish to retain his power of thought. Although it may be thought desirable to give drugs orally, nausea and vomiting can cause problems, and the effect of giving an anti-emetic can be tried before resorting to injections. The success at controlling pain achieved by those who specialise in the care of the dying is not merely due to giving large quantities of drugs, but to their skill in assessing all the patient's physical and mental problems, and meeting them.

Simple analgesics

Aspirin is most effective when used for reducing pain in muscles, bones and ligaments. It will reduce the temperature of a feverish patient, and has some effect on inflammation. Its success with headache is perhaps due to the fact that many headaches are caused by tension in the structures overlying the skull.

Long continued administration may lead to chronic blood loss from slow oozing from the intestinal tract, and sometimes frank melaena occurs. Asthmatics should not take aspirin, to which they are often sensitive, and it interacts with many other drugs.

Aspirin is quite effective for pain in bones due to secondary malignant disease, though a stronger drug will eventually be needed. The most efficient and least irritating form is the soluble one.

Paracetamol (Panadol) is a mild analgesic useful in circumstances similar to those in which aspirin is used.

Aspirin, paracetamol and other drugs are sometimes combined in mixtures, but the use of these in terminal pain is not always advisable, since it is desirable to know the effect of each component when dosage has to be adjusted.

More powerful drugs

All the drugs described in this section act centrally, i.e. on the brain. Some are comparatively mild (e.g. codeine, dihydrocodeine). Some have been synthesised by pharmaceutical companies in the hope of producing a drug with the pain-relieving properties of morphine, but without its addictive features, and some of its other unwanted side-effects. The milder analgesics will be described first, and finally morphine and diamorphine, which will very often be needed in the management of those with malignant disease in its last phases. None of the synthetic drugs can rival these two in relieving physical pain and distress, but some suit particular circumstances.

Codeine is only about a quarter as effective an analgesic as morphine, but less liable to cause respiratory depression and constipation. It is very widely used to relieve moderate pain, sometimes with aspirin. Linctus codeine is a good cough suppressant. It is usually given by mouth; if injections have to be used, something stronger is preferred.

Dihydrocodeine (DF118) is said to have fewer side-effects than codeine, but is constipating, and has not displaced codeine in public favour.

Pethidine acts mostly on smooth muscle, as in the intestine and uterus, and while it is very effective when used for its best purpose, it does not have a great deal of use in terminal care. It has little hypnotic effect, so does not calm the fearful patient.

It can be given by mouth or intramuscular injection.

Methadone also lacks the calming effect of the opiates, but it is an effective analgesic by mouth or by injection. Dependence occurs less often than with morphine, and it is often used in treating morphine or heroin (diamorphine) addicts. Its use for the dying appears to be decreasing.

Phenazocine (Narphen) is a synthetic developed in the hope that it would be as effective as, but less addictive, than morphine.

Pentazocine (Fortral) is a related drug. Both of these are quite widely used, but hopes that they are not addictive have been disappointed, and there are a number of people who are dependent on pentazocine, and these include hospital staff. Nausea, vomiting and dizziness are unwanted side-effects, and the elderly are prone to hallucinations.

Dipipanone is found to be effective by some prescribers. Diconal is a combination of dipipanone with an anti-emetic, cyclizine, and is helpful when nausea has to be controlled.

Oxycodone pectinate has a longer action than many analgesics, and is popular for the use of those in pain at home. A dose in the evening may be sufficient to prevent pain throughout the night.

Dextromoramide (Palfium) is less sedative than morphine, and is quite widely used in the oral treatment of terminal pain.

Dextropropoxyphene is effective for moderate pain; very large doses may produce mental symptoms. In combination with paracetamol (Distalgesic) it is a very popular analgesic with a marked calming effect, but there is an increasing problem of drug abuse in connection with it. As a general rule, compound analgesics are not suitable for the terminally ill, though many forms exist. It is desirable to keep prescribing simple, so as to be able to identify quickly the cause of any untoward reaction or side effect.

New synthetic analgesics are formulated and put on the

market regularly. Nurses who are interested in the drugs they give to their patients (and this should mean all of us), should consult the British National Formulary, which is kept in most wards and all nursing libraries. The publishers hope to produce a new edition twice a year, so that up to date information is always available.

The central action of these drugs mean that they are cough suppressants as well as analgesics, and that they tend to produce nausea, which may need countering by an anti-emetic.

Anti-inflammatory drugs like phenylbutazone and indomethacin which are used in the treatment of rheumatoid arthritis may be effective in reducing the pain of bony metastases.

Steroids also have a place in the management of bone pain, and the euphoric effect they have is invaluable in keeping up the spirits. Headache due to increasing intracranial pressure is better treated by high-dose steroids such as dexamethasone than by opiates.

Morphine and Diamorphine

In general hospitals, when patients have been dying with some painful condition, there has been traditionally a reluctance to use morphine until late in the illness. It was felt that people rapidly became dependent, demanding bigger and more frequent doses, exhibiting personality changes and passing into a state wretched for themselves, their families, and their attendants. Doctors and nurses in hospices and similar places have shown that this unfortunate result is a management failure, and can be avoided. It results from treating a fearful patient with a rigid inadequate schedule of morphine by injection. People can live a relatively normal life for long periods on a well planned prescription.

Morphine is the principal alkaloid of opium, and its many properties make it one of the most important drugs available. Its principal uses are:
  1. To relieve pain, for which it is excellent.

2. To produce calm and a sense of wellbeing (euphoria) in tense and frightened people.

It is these two actions that make it so effective in (e.g.) coronary heart disease, as well as in the care of the dying.

3. It controls cough.

4. It is a good indirect haemostat, helping to control gastrointestinal bleeding by sedating the patient and reducing peristalsis.

5. It is excellent for the severe breathlessness of acute left ventricular heart failure.

6. It is widely used before operation for its calming effect, as well as afterwards to relieve pain.

It is easy to judge when someone has had morphine by the dreamy euphoria, and by the contracted pupils. There are more important side-effects to be considered. Constipation is very common, and must be actively treated and prevented, as described in the section on bowel management (p. 31), or serious physical consequences may follow. Nausea and vomiting may occur, and necessitate giving an anti-emetic. Depression of the respiratory centre is a well known morphine effect, which can be useful when controlling breathlessness in the dying.

Morphine is much less well absorbed by mouth than it is by injection, but nevertheless it should be given by mouth to the dying. Injections, especially repeated injections, are an ordeal, and giving a series of intramuscular injections to an emaciated patient is a trial not only for him but for his nurse. It is often possible to care for a patient up to a very late stage with oral morphine.

The dose will depend on how much the patient needs to prevent pain occurring, and although over days or weeks it will often be necessary to raise the dose, this is not a troublesome feature when the drug is given by mouth. In general, the interval should be about four hours. Regularity is of the utmost importance but there is no rigid timetable, and the patient is never told that he must wait for his analgesic. If he is in pain after a shorter interval, it is an indication that the dose should be increased.

A very well known mixture containing morphine is Morphine and Cocaine Elixir BPC. It contains a little alcohol. 'Brompton Cocktail' was a term widely used about a mixture of these three ingredients, but this is a popular name, not a definite prescription. The amount of morphine can be varied by the prescriber, and many doctors prefer to omit the cocaine. Other elixirs in the National Formulary contain chloropromazine, to allay anxiety and reduce the risk of vomiting. Morphine suppositories are useful when the patient tolerates morphine poorly by mouth, and it is desired to avoid injections. Suppositories are comparatively little used in this country except as laxatives, but in Europe they are widely used. It is thought that it is a rather undignified way of giving a medicine, but many patients can and do put suppositories in place themselves. They can be useful in care at home. Morphine Slow Release Tablets are effective for up to twelve hours, and are also valuable for patients at home.

To give a drug to control anxiety may not be the treatment required. There may be an element of falsity in the situation if relatives or the doctor feel that the patient must not learn the truth about his situation. To keep up a facade of optimism in such conditions about recovery, when it is clear to the patient that no such recovery is happening, may cause acute anxiety. The question of how and when a patient is given the opportunity to learn the truth is discussed in Chapter 6. It is not suggested that the knowledge that one's condition is terminal will automatically take away anxiety; there are many elements in such anxiety, but giving an antidepressant is only one way of reducing it.

Diamorphine (Heroin). The medical use of diamorphine is legal in Great Britain, but prohibited in many countries because of its dangers as a drug of addiction. Banning the use of diamorphine by doctors has had no effect, however, on the illicit traffic, because contraband heroin does not come from legal manufacturing processes.

The actions of diamorphine closely resemble those of morphine. Weight for weight it is more powerful than morphine, which explains why it is more popular with drug peddlers— it is less bulky and so more profitable. Although some doctors think very highly of it, in the case of the dying, diamorphine has no advantages over morphine when taken by mouth. It is very valuable in those cases for whom injections become necessary, since the effective volume of diamorphine is smaller than that of morphine, and so causes less discomfort in administration.

Other drugs. Relief of pain by analgesics takes precedence over most procedures, but it must not be thought that some one who is receiving adequate pain relief will necessarily be free from distress or anxiety. The patient suffers from impending bereavement, just as relatives do, and may have acute fears about business, or children, or how a surviving spouse will cope emotionally or financially. An open and free discussion without dissimulation is helpful, but a tranquilliser may be required, like chloropromazine or diazepam, if the mood is agitated. For depression, there is a variety of drugs; among the tricyclic group, imipramine or amitriptyline can be used.

The drugs used in the relief of pain in the dying have been discussed bearing in mind someone with severe pain from malignant disease. There are, however, many other causes of pain, and these can also afflict the dying. The pain of mouth ulcers, or pressure sores may over-ride all other problems in the patient's mind. These it is hoped to prevent or cure by standard nursing means. Headache, indigestion or piles can cause great distress. This is a good example of how a personal nursing plan, well thought out and executed, will benefit the individual.

Sleeplessness may be less of a problem when pain and anxiety have been dealt with. The use of small quantities of alcohol last thing at night for the elderly has already been alluded to, and a simple sedative like nitrazepam (Mogadon) may be given.

Nausea and vomiting are complications of opiate therapy, and they are also complications of some fatal conditions. It is very commonly caused by constipation, which must be prevented. There are many anti-emetic drugs; metoclopramide (Maxolon) is an effective one; if it cannot be retained by mouth, cyclizine by injection can be tried. Simple nursing measures should not be omitted; small quantities of ice-cold fluid can be tried, and effervescent liquids like tonic water may be liked. Prescribing should be kept as simple as possible. Multiple drugs interact with each other, and make it difficult to understand the clinical picture. As soon as the reason for giving a drug no longer exists, it should be cancelled.

Nurses from non-specialist hospitals attending courses or study days on the care of the dying often ask what they can do when doctors are slow or unwilling to raise medication for increasing pain, or to make a change. Whether it is true or no, it is evidently a feeling that nurses experience. It must be remembered that nurses spend more time with their dying patients than doctors do, and so are more vulnerable to their expressed needs. Nurses are not more humane than doctors, but they have longer time in which to observe symptoms.

The answer to the question is that nurses should draw the doctor's attention to the patient's needs, should ring him up for advice when the patient is in pain and no drug is due, and ask him to visit. When he becomes aware of the nature and extent of the problem a helpful response can be expected.

5

Devising and giving individual care: the nursing process

In the last two chapters, attention has been given to the symptoms that may arise in terminal illness, and the nursing techniques that are used in preventing or relieving them. A good knowledge of the events that may occur is an essential part of the nurse's skill, which enables her to forestall troubles, and good practical knowledge permits her to give effective care. But acquiring such knowledge and ability is only a part of the nurse's equipment for giving truly professional service. We do not care for cancer, for pain, for depression, but for people who are afflicted with such conditions, and who react to them and judge their importance in a completely individual way.

To illustrate how the needs of people with a similar diagnostic label may have quite different needs to be met by their nurses, we can consider the stories of two women.

Joan was a doctor, 52 years old, in general practice with a partner in Dorset. She was unmarried, living alone in a comfortable house which she owned in a small town. Her nearest relatives were a sister, and a married brother, both of whom lived in London and with whom she was on close and cordial terms. She enjoyed her work, and was a popular and hardworking general practitioner with many friends.

In June 1978 she noticed that she had a lump in her left breast. Though small, it was hard and painless, and she felt at once that it must be malignant. Her doctor confirmed her fears, and a week later she entered hospital for mastectomy and a postoperative course of radiotherapy. Her progress was uneventful, and after convalescence she returned to her practice. Her health remained apparently good for the next year, but then a lump appeared in her left axilla. The surgeon confirmed that it was a secondary growth, and also noticed that her liver was enlarged. She was consulted about treatment, and agreed to radiotherapy and asked about prognosis. She was told that early recurrence was not a hopeful sign, but that her condition remained treatable.

She went home to consult with her partner about practice details, and to talk with her family about where she should live if she became incapable of coping on her own. This decision was not urgent; she had domestic help, and many friends both medical and lay who called regularly and on whom she could depend.

Her present admission came six months later. She now had headaches and dizziness, revealed by brain scan to be due to secondaries, and she had difficulty in walking. She was given further radiotherapy to the skull, and prescribed cytotoxic drugs and prednisolone. Her condition began to deteriorate quite rapidly, and it was clear that her illness would soon be fatal. The prednisolone had a distinctly euphoric effect, and she remained cheerful, discussing her symptoms and their causes with her nurses and doctors.

Joan's physical state presented no unusual problems to the nurses, but she was a highly intelligent woman, professionally well informed and able to interpret the meaning of new symptoms. Though cheerful and kindly to everyone, she soon became impatient with euphemisms, or optimistic statements that were not founded on fact. For some time she felt that she might hope to resume limited activity for a time, and she took interest and pains with her appearance and toilet, wearing a hair piece to hide her hair loss, liking to keep her nails polished, and to use her usual perfume and talcum powder. One of her problems was the number of friends who wanted to call; they believed they were sustaining her, but in fact she was upholding them and gradually she said goodbye and they were asked not to call without phoning, so that it was possible to confine her callers to her family.

The second patient had a similar diagnosis on admission, but this was the only way in which Joan resembled Anne.

Anne B was a married woman, 66 years old, living with her husband, a retired office worker, in a London flat. They were childless. The husband had had a mild coronary illness two years previously but had no symptoms now, except a little anxiety about his heart. It was twelve years since Anne had had any serious health problem, when she had had a mastectomy for a growth in the right breast. Since then there had been no sign of recurrence, and she had done the work of her flat and lived a normal social life. She had some problems over sleep, and she ascribed this to the noise of traffic at night. She smoked about twelve cigarettes a day, and had a slight persistent cough. She would have liked to stop smoking, but felt it calmed her nerves.

A month ago she began to get severe pain in her lumbar spine, and went to see her doctor, who prescribed an analgesic, rest and local warmth. He noticed the cough and the question of smoking was raised. He asked her to come again in a week's time, and when she returned the pain was even worse. She was fatigued, and losing weight. Her doctor sent her to hospital for X-ray. This showed that she had secondary deposits in the spine, and also growths in the chest, which contained a considerable amount of fluid. She was admitted to a ward at once for assessment. As far as she knew, she had lumbago and a smoker's cough. Her husband was told that she had widespread malignant disease, and that although treatment would be given, the outlook was poor. She returned home under the care of the oncological department. Her husband was able to look after her needs, as she was not bed ridden.

These stories concern women who both have metastasis from breast cancer and are in terminal illness. Both have received the same kind of medical treatment — operation, radiotherapy and chemotherapy — but it will at once be seen that their personal and social needs at this stage are quite different. Joan is fully aware of the nature of her illness, and able to interpret any symptoms that arise. Anne does not as yet know the true nature of her illness. Joan has no dependents, but has loving supporting relatives. Anne has a husband with a history of a heart attack, and no close family ties. Each will have different needs, and different expectations. Joan's brother and sister will be grief-stricken; Anne's husband will be living alone, attending to his own needs, and coping with anxiety about his heart as well as with his bereavement.

Ever since skilled professional nursing began, the most skilled nurses have given care that is tailored to each patient. In order to ensure that all learners are taught how to reach the best standards, and that all patients receive personally devised care, a formal method of planning is required.

The Nursing Process is a method with a well researched theoretical base, and as such is often described in formal terms which some nurses may find difficult to understand, and which leads them to feel that the 'Process' is of theoretical rather than practical value. Before discussing and illustrating it, it can be described in simple terms that show that this is not so. The steps in planning and executing a nursing care plan for an individual patient are as follows.

1. Find out as many facts as possible about the patient and his family as are relevant to nursing this particular person well, and helping his family. This relevant information must be written down, so that it is available to all the nurses on day and night duty.

2. On the basis of this information, plan the nursing care for this patient. Specific and definite nursing goals should be set, and written down.

3. Give the nursing care that will help us reach the goals we have set.

4. Judge regularly how successful we have been in giving good care, and use this knowledge in improving our skills which we shall use in nursing other patients.

Each of these steps can be examined in detail and applied to the care of a particular patient in his last illness, or to his family.

Assessment

When a patient is admitted to hospital, the doctor interviews him as soon as possible and takes a medical history, and from the information he gains he makes or confirms the diagnosis and decides on treatment. If we believe that nursing is a distinct profession in its own right, with special skills to contribute, we will also believe that we must take a nursing history, from which we will be enabled to find the patient's special problems, and to solve those that fall within our scope. The process of discovering these problems and needs through a nursing history is termed 'assessment'. It is only through possession of facts that we will be able to see needs and perhaps hope to meet them, and it is only by a systematic and professional approach that we shall gain this knowledge.

Let us suppose that the afternoon report is being taken on a surgical ward by the sister from her staff, and that all the learners are listening, and taking note of changes of treatment or condition. Patient allocation is increasingly being used to organise nursing care. This means that each nurse gives a report on the patients she has looked after and the qualified nurse adds information or corrects the nurse as necessary. The nurse might say 'Mr Smith; no change', and this would be accepted as a kind of shorthand for the fact that there has been no change of treatment for Mr Smith, but of course all of us change from one day to another. Looking at the admission list for the next day, she reads 'Arthur T., carcinoma of rectum'. A new student might ask 'What is the treatment for carcinoma of rectum?'. We do not treat carcinoma but the person who is afflicted by it, since cancer only exists when it affects someone. But this shorthand again is well understood, and sister might speak of abdomino-perineal resection of rectum, of the severity of the operation, of the effects of colostomy on life in the community after discharge.

When Arthur T. is admitted next day, taking a nursing history may reveal that his problems are entirely different from those which his surgical diagnosis has suggested, and which merely tells us the condition from which he is going to die.

This is the nursing history of Arthur T. obtained mostly from his sister, and partly from observing Mr T.

Mr T. is 74, and has lived for many years with his sister and brother-in-law. This is his first admission to hospital, and indeed the first time he has been away from his sister.

Six months ago he began to have pain, especially on defaecation, and to pass blood with the stools. His doctor found he had carcinoma of rectum, and that it had reached an inoperable stage.

Mr T. is mentally retarded; he cannot read or write. He has also been an epileptic all his life. Fits are fairly well controlled by epanutin and phenobarbitone, but he sometimes has an attack at night. He becomes restless, breathing is stertorous, he fights for breath, may scream, and becomes very agitated. His sister is able to reassure him and calm him down. He is unaware of his diagnosis, and almost certainly incapable of realising its implications.

He gets pain in the right side of the abdomen, and although he does not usually complain, he groans and grimaces during an attack. He has a bowel action every two or three hours, and sometimes this helps to ease the pain. He loses blood in the stools. He has been prescribed pethidine tablets, but these are no longer fully effective.

Some of his habits and tastes, that are of importance to the nurses in caring for Mr T., and his very special needs are as follows.

Food. Most of his teeth have been extracted. Despite this, his food does not have to be soft, and he enjoys his meals, though his appetite is not as good as it was.

Sleep. He slept well until recently, when he had to get up because of his diarrhoea.

Drinks. He likes most fluids, but will not drink from a feeder. He takes sugar in coffee, but not in tea.

Excretion. He has no problems with passing urine. His bowel habit has been described.

Exercise. He has lost a good deal of weight from muscle wasting, and is now unable to walk without support.

Hygiene. He used to enjoy a shower, but for the last two weeks his sister has washed him in bed.

Religion. Non-conformist. He has a simple Christian faith. He enjoys hymn-singing and television programmes like *Songs of Praise*. He would like to attend the hospital chapel, his sister says, if it could be managed.

Hobbies. He keeps 'notebooks' in which he likes to scribble with coloured pencils. He likes looking at picture books and listening to music. When there is no television he will quite happily look at the test card and listen to the music.

Mood. On admission he was uneasy and anxious, especially when his sister left, although she told him she would call again to see him in the evening. However, it proved easy to reassure

him. Smiles, and a few words soon helped him to settle in
cheerfully.

Family. His sister was deeply anxious about how he would cope
without her, and is keen to give any information that would
help the nurses in caring for him. It was also evident that she
would miss caring for him herself, heavy and constant as the
task was. She was more concerned with his happiness and
comfort now than his forthcoming death; she had often worried
about what would happen to him if she were to become
incapacitated or die.

It will be seen that speculations about operations and colostomy and a good prognosis are irrelevant. It will also be seen
that he and his sister have many needs that nurses can hope to
meet, once they have become aware of them.

Taking a nursing history must be systematic. It need not be
unduly time-consuming, but it will almost certainly be
cumulative, as more information becomes available from the
patient and his relatives, and as the medical and nursing
picture develops. The necessity for recording it, so that all
nurses may know it, becomes clear. It will certainly be necessary to have some kind of form to guide the nurse, and to
indicate to her what is relevant. This form will vary from one
speciality to another, but in general these sorts of headings are
appropriate.

Registry data. The patient's name, address and similar
details are already available from the admission sheet.
Although these are required for the nursing history, there
seems no good reason for asking the patient for them rather
than transferring them.

Reasons for admission. The history of the present illness will
again be in the doctor's notes, and need not be repeated in
detail, though it is a good means of starting communication
with the patient, since most people like talking about their
illness. The reason for not calling this section 'Present illness'
is that the nurse wants to know what the patient sees as the
reason for admission. For instance, Joan knew she was coming into hospital for the treatment of metastases; Anne
thought she was going to have her lumbago and her cough

treated. It would not have been very useful to ask Arthur why he was in hospital; it would only have confused that simple soul. In general, it is always useful to know what the patient sees as the most important symptom, since if that is not relieved he will not be satisfied. In the case of the dying, fear of pain is the most usual symptom, though sometimes the dying become concerned with rather marginal matters, such as lack of appetite, rather than face more important topics.

Personal information. These are the facts about the patient's habits on religion, eating, drinking, sleeping, bowel habit, hobbies, family relations and problems. Looking back at Arthur's history it will be seen how important this information is in allowing the nurses to give small nursing attentions that will make him feel at ease.

Psychophysical state. Nurses understand this section well; they are used to making records and observations, and these assume real importance when they are to form the basis of a care plan. It is convenient to consider these records by systems.

(a) *Circulatory system*, e.g. pulse rate and rhythm; blood pressure.

(b) *Respiratory system*, e.g. rate and character of breathing; cough; sputum; presence of dyspnoea or orthopnoea.

(c) *Musculoskeletal system*, e.g. paralysis; weakness; wasting; the amount of walking the patient can undertake, if any; oedema.

(d) *Special senses*. Hearing and sight are the most important in maintaining communication.

(e) *Digestive system*, e.g. weight; wasting; constipation; diarrhoea; vomiting; signs of dehydration, appetite. One of the last pleasures that the dying can enjoy is often small appetizing meals.

(f) *Genitourinary system*, e.g. output, frequency, continence. A symptom like incontinence may be a grave problem to the dying with the loss of personal dignity entailed.

(g) *Skin*, e.g. nutritional and hygienic state; signs of impending or actual pressure sores. A pressure sore and its attendant pain may be a great trial to a patient in a final illness.

(h) *Central nervous system*, e.g. level of consciousness; paralysis.

(i) *Mental state*. Any of the reactions mentioned in the chapter on psychological reactions (p. 58) may be dominant at one stage or another of the last illness.

(j) *Planned medical treatment*. This especially relates, in the case of the dying, to the prescription of analgesic drugs, so that the doctor's treatment will generate an important section of nursing care.

In writing up the assessment, an effort should be made only to record facts and not opinions, and to keep the account relevant. If the history becomes too verbose, this system of planning care becomes tedious and eventually discredited.

Planning Nursing Care

When Mr T. was only a diagnosis on admission card, we had some knowledge about how his condition might be treated, but none at all about Mr T's problems. Now that we have a nursing history the variety and magnitude of his problems can be realised, and therefore an informed effort made to summarise these and decide what action the nurses can take about them.

A list is made of his needs, and of the goals that the nurses might set themselves with regard to them. This list may well lengthen as more information becomes available, or his condition changes. Some may prove impossible to attain and must be changed. For instance, we notice that Mr T. has problems in walking through muscular weakness, and set ourselves the goal of improving his gait until he can walk unaided. Soon we realise that his weakness is due to his advancing disease, and that he needs no more than to be helped into a chair near his bed, if he so wishes.

We shall almost certainly aim to keep the skin over the pressure areas intact, perhaps by four hourly turning and the use of a fleece beneath the buttocks. If signs of redness nevertheless appear we shall not abandon our goal, but use further effort to achieve it, perhaps by two hourly turning, and the use of a large-cell ripple mattress. His problems are set out, and the objectives we set ourselves about each one. Following that, come the details of how we are to achieve this.

Nursing Problems	*Objectives of Care*
His first experience of hospital; he is anxious and frightened.	He will settle into hospital quickly and happily.

Nursing care. He is reassured by being spoken to when a nurse passes, orientated to his surroundings, given his own belongings, smiled at. His sister and brother-in-law are encouraged to visit regularly, and are asked what else we can do for him.

Nursing Problems	*Objectives of care*
He has right-sided abdominal pain due to his cancer.	The pain shall be controlled.

Nursing care. Pain-relieving drugs are given regularly as prescribed, and the effect observed. Conferring with the doctor may lead to modification of the dose. As Mr T. very rarely complains verbally, he is watched for tension, unease or grimaces.

Nursing Problems	*Objectives of care*
He has diarrhoea by day and also by night, which disturbs his rest.	Bowel actions should be 2 or 3 by day, none by night.

Nursing care. Control of pain may decrease bowel irritability. He is helped to a commode when necessary, and reassured that it is always immediately available. Morphine mixtures may help prevent diarrhoea as well as relieving pain. A sedative at night would not normally be needed.

Nursing Problems	*Objectives of care*
He has epilepsy.	Fits should be prevented.

Nursing care. The anti-convulsive drugs ordered are given and

Mr T. observed, especially at night for fits. Should these occur the dose of his drugs may be adjusted. He is reassured by the night nurse, as he was by his sister at home. A padded spoon might be kept on the locker if tongue biting happens.

Nursing Problems	*Objectives of Care*
He is mentally retarded.	He shall function happily within his limitations.

Nursing care. Life shall be simplified for him; he is not asked to make decisions or burdened with information he cannot understand. He is encouraged to keep his 'notebooks', and picture books may be offered from the librarian. He can listen with headphones to the radio and look at television if he wants to. The non-conformist chaplain will call, and should be told of Mr T's limits. He is to be treated with respect; his sister has found him a loving and lovable companion for many years.

Nursing Problems	*Objectives of Care*
He cannot attend to his personal hygiene because of weakness.	To maintain personal hygiene.

Nursing care. He is regularly bathed in bed. His anal area may become sore due to diarrhoea, and soft paraffin can be applied. He is to have a fleece beneath the buttocks, and to be turned four hourly if he is not active himself. He may brush his teeth with supervision.

Nursing Problems	*Objectives of Care*
His illness is a terminal one.	To ensure a peaceful end.

Nursing care. Once his pain is controlled and diarrhoea lessened, he should be comfortable. He is not able to understand death and no effort should be made to explain it.

Nursing Problems	Objectives of Care
His sister is full of anxiety about him.	She and her husband shall accept his loss.

Nursing care. His sister is encouraged to talk to the nurses and to the chaplain. She is praised for the marvellous care she has given, and reminded that Mr T. is fortunate if he does not have to face life without her.

Giving Care

Putting the nursing care plan into action involves setting out to achieve particular aims, and not merely doing a series of tasks. The nurse can use her judgement in varying the means of achieving her aims, if one method is not successful. There is no room for vague instructions like 'Give all general nursing care', or 'Treat pressure areas'. Nurses know their aims, and devise the best means of fulfilling them.

Evaluation

This means, judging the results of our efforts to reach our nursing objectives. This judgement should if possible be based on observable facts. Evaluation in nursing of any particular person is an on-going affair; we regularly review our aims and see if we are reaching them, if we must change our methods, or abandon some particular goal. For instance, keeping Mr T. pain-free is a major goal, and our success or absence of it reviewed constantly. A change of drug or an increase of dose may be necessary; it is never a goal to be abandoned.

Mr T. adjusted well to his move to hospital, and his sister was much relieved by his good adjustment and his lack of pain. About a fortnight after admission, his condition deteriorated rapidly, probably due to internal bleeding, and he died peacefully, in the company of his sister and brother-in-law.

Final evaluation of the nursing care that Mr T. received showed that the nursing objectives had been well met. The ward sister could congratulate her team on their success in dealing with some unusual problems. In particular, Mr T's sister had been able to see that his end had been peaceful, and that her care of him had continued up to his death. The nurses also learned a lesson. They had seen that an elderly, mentally retarded person can inspire love and respect, and that they themselves could find fulfilment in devising a personal plan for him, and carrying it out successfully in his last illness.

6

Understanding the feelings of the dying

The aim of this chapter is to give the nurse some insight into the feelings which a patient may experience when he is dying and how these feelings may be manifested in his words and behaviour. It suggests ways of helping the patient with these feelings and with coming to terms with death. Each patient is an individual and his dying is a unique experience for him. No one is able to tell him exactly what it will be like or how he will feel. It is a new phase of his life which will eventually end. The nurse's support and understanding at such a time in his life is of great importance.

The emotional needs of the dying are less clearly defined than physical needs. They involve the patient's knowledge that he is dying, his reactions to death, his personal belief about death and his relationship with his family, friends and colleagues. Each person brings his own character and personality, his relationship with others and his past experiences to the way in which he faces death and therefore his emotional needs are varied and complex. It is important that the nurse uses the information in this chapter as guidelines only to the emotional support she gives to the dying, and not as definitive answers to complicated emotional problems.

Knowledge About Death

How does anyone discover that he is dying? In one sense, he has known it all his adult life. All of us, except followers of a few religious sects, recognise that our life on this earth has a natural span that ends in death. In youth we give little thought to it, but as we grow older grandparents die, then parents, and at last our contemporaries, and the subject becomes of more personal immediacy. Listening to and thinking about people's hopes or fears about death, it becomes clear that most people are more concerned about the last stages of their life than their final departure. They fear inactivity, loneliness, loss of independence, suffering pain, and being a burden to others. When in the last stages they realise that death is near, they may also realise that their fears about terminal illness are groundless.

Some people of course die suddenly as the result of an accident, or a fatal heart attack, or do not recognise that they are dying. Others may lapse into unconsciousness as a result, for instance, of a stroke or a severe injury, and are unaware of the approaching end. Young children are unable to appreciate what is happening, though they often seem to know that they will not get better.

The rest arrive at the point of death more slowly. Some may have had conditions like kidney or liver failure, which treatment has controlled for some time, but which is now no longer effective. Some may know that they have cancer, and have had more or less lengthy treatment by surgery, radiotherapy and drugs. Others may have very little insight into the cause of their illness, but recognise its seriousness. Many are elderly, and accept their failing powers at the end of a long life. Some cannot accept that their illness is fatal, and look desperately for other forms of treatment to prolong their lives. Every report of a new treatment for malignant disease brings floods of enquiries, and every unorthodox kind of therapy can find adherents.

Not only, therefore, are there many categories of dying patients, but each consists of a host of individuals, all different in their natures, responsibilities, families and circumstances. It can be seen that there is no simple universally applicable answer to the question, Should a person be told of his approaching death? The present trend of public opinion is for more information from doctors and nurses, and to believe that patients have a right to knowledge about themselves. But since it is the doctors and nurses who possess this information, their beliefs about what they should release, or to whom, is paramount.

The usual answer that professionals return when asked what information should be given to the dying patient, is that it depends on each individual. This is blameless, but not very informative. The doctor becomes the judge of what is best for each one, but his answer will be guided by his own beliefs. The research done on this topic in the United States and this country indicates that there is quite a high level of unwillingness among nurses and general practitioners to tell the truth, and that more than half would like to give some hope. (See *Life Before Death* (1973). Ann Cartwright, Lisbeth Hockey and John Anderson. Routledge and Kegan Paul.)

The following story shows that a peaceful and happy end may be achieved without telling the patient of his approaching death.

Twelve years ago Mr S. had a total laryngectomy for carcinoma. At that time his wife said that he was not told that the operation was for cancer, and Mr S. claimed that he did not know the reason for such radical surgery. However, since then he had been well except for the occasional chest infection. He had also mastered oesophageal speech and it was easy to understand him. Then he developed a nagging pain in his right wrist; at first he thought he had strained a muscle while gardening, but when the pain did not go away, and in fact got worse, he decided to consult his general practitioner. His doctor could find no cause for his pain on examination and therefore referred him to hospital for further investigations. An X-ray of his right wrist was suggestive of a bony metastasis. This was confirmed by a bone scan which also revealed other metastases in his right upper arm and rib cage, presumably from the primary carcinoma of larynx. When Mrs S. was seen by the consultant, she was adamant that her husband should not be told of the cancer and its spread. The consultant in outpatients agreed to this in the first instance and prescribed Distalgesic for Mr S. to help the pain.

A month after seeing the consultant Mr S. was admitted to a medical ward with a chest infection and increasing pain in his right wrist. He was a tall, thin seventy-year-old man who was meticulous about his personal hygiene. He cared for his permanent tracheostomy himself and wore a small white bib over the opening. His wife was petite, timid and very anxious about her husband. She reiterated again to the ward sister that her husband was not to be told about his diagnosis, although the sister did explain gently that it might be necessary to tell him if he asked outright. Mr S. settled down quickly in the ward and received physiotherapy and antibiotics for his chest infection. Indomethacin was prescribed regularly with Distalgesic, and this proved an effective combination to control his pain. The nurses ensured that he always had the Indomethacin with meals or a glass of milk in order to prevent stomach irritation.

Mr S. was a quiet man who at first asked very little about his condition. However he did talk a lot about the meaning of his own life as he felt that it had not been worthwhile. He had not contributed to society in a dramatic way. He had only one daughter who was happily married and living in Canada with her husband. She had a highly successful career, but no children. Mr S. admitted that he was disappointed not to have grandchildren. He sometimes asked the nurses why they bothered with 'an old man like me'. The nurses were able to reassure him that everyone was worth 'bothering' about. Mr S. was given several opportunities by the medical and senior nursing staff to ask about his condition and treatment, as some of them felt that he wanted to know his diagnosis. However, the nearest he ever came to admitting that he was aware of his prognosis was to say that he knew that the pain in his wrist could not be cured completely, but only alleviated by tablets.

After two weeks in hospital Mr S. was discharged home to his wife. However, he was back after ten days with another chest infection. He was also weaker this time and his wife felt unable to cope at home. In view of his general deterioration Mrs S. was advised to contact her daughter in Canada who decided to fly over a few days later to be with her parents. Mr S. was disappointed to be back in hospital again so soon, but relieved to be on the same ward where he knew most of the nurses and some of the patients. This time he found it more difficult to expectorate his sputum, and therefore the nurses sometimes gave him tracheal suction. A suction machine was plugged in by his bedside with the necessary equipment, and only used for Mr S.

The pain in Mr S's wrist was worse so it was decided to commence Diamorphine Elixir 5 mg in a gin and orange base. This was given regularly every four hours and was effective in controlling Mr S's pain.

Mr S. was delighted to see his daughter when she arrived from Canada, but tears came to his eyes on her first visit to the ward. Perhaps he realised that as her trip to England was unexpected he must be very ill. However, he never spoke about this to either his family or the nursing staff.

Mr S. gradually became weaker but up until his last day he insisted on walking out to the bathroom. He was very unsteady on his feet but determined to keep going. The nurses respected this by helping him to the bathroom and letting him retain his independence. At times he became very angry and impatient when the nurses offered to help him to wash or shave. Some of the junior nurses were upset by this and therefore the problem was discussed at report time with all the nurses. As a result, it was decided to respect Mr S's wishes, and let him only wash his hands and face if this was what he wanted. The sister made it clear that she would not criticise the nurse caring for him if Mr S. did not have a complete wash every day.

Mr S. never talked openly about dying but the nurses felt he knew, and they respected his wish not to talk about it. On his last afternoon he had to be carried back to bed from the bathroom as he was too weak to walk. Tucked up in bed, he fell asleep with his wife on one side and his daughter on the other. He never woke again as he died three hours later peacefully and in the dignified way in which he had lived.

The question as to whether relatives should be told is less controversial. Most believe that the relatives should know. This will put a strain on the family and create a false situation if the patient is not told as well.

In general, hospice staff who deal only with the dying believe that the patient must not be told untruths, must be given full opportunity to discuss his illness, and should decide himself when to ask if he is dying.

If someone in the last stages of his illness is transferred to a hospice or to another ward, the doctor who admits him and examines him should at the end of the interview ask the patient if he has any questions, and should sit beside him and wait without hurry. Some people will say 'No thank you', and these are not yet ready to acknowledge that their illness is terminal. Some will ask quite plainly if they are going to die, and should be given a plain sympathetic, but truthful answer. The next question then will be, 'How long have I got left?' This is a question that must be carefully treated; if the answer is hours or days it can usually be fairly accurately assessed. If it is likely to be weeks or months a precise answer cannot be given.

Sometimes a patient asks less definite questions. 'Can you do anything for me?' can always be answered in the affirmative. We can control and prevent pain, or relieve troublesome symptoms. We must always be alert for meanings that the patient is trying to convey. 'When shall I be able to go home?' may mean that he has little idea that his illness is terminal, or alternatively that he would like to be at home when he dies. 'How long shall I be here?' may mean, 'How soon shall I be discharged', or, on the other hand, 'How much longer have I got to live?'

The staff and the chaplains should all be aware of the patient's state of knowledge because the nurses will certainly be asked further questions. A patient who has been told he is going to die will subsequently ask his nurse, seeking confirmation or perhaps even hoping for denial. Some who have been told manage to put the thought out of their minds, and do not mention it again. Though a truthful answer must be given to questions it can be softened by not revealing the whole truth. For example, if the patient asks, 'Am I going to die?', the nurse may reply, 'I don't think that you are going to get better' rather than a stark reply of 'Yes'. Unless honest answers are given to a patient, a trustful relationship cannot be built up which is so necessary for a patient to give him support and care to the end. It is equally important that a person's hope in the future is not taken away or he will become utterly despondent.

A patient's insight into his condition does not only come from what he is told directly by members of the caring team. He has his own past experience of others who have died, his observations of his own condition and other people's behaviour towards him. All these give him clues that he may be dying. A person who does not ask questions about his illness may not have been given the opportunity to ask, or he may be afraid that he will be given platitudes and not the truth. Evasion of truth that a person is dying is a protective mechanism for the doctor or nurse who may not feel able to cope with the patient's reaction to the news. The doctor may view the patient's coming death as a failure on his part to be able to prevent it with drugs or other medical treatment. Nevertheless, the caring team must put these personal feelings aside and deal honestly with the dying patient's questions. In this way a trusting relationship is gradually built up.

Not all patients do want to have the information that they are dying put into words. Some instinctively know it or have been told indirectly by non-verbal cues from relatives or staff. As nurses we are not always aware that our behaviour can tell a patient that he is dying. We may be more painstaking over our care of him compared to others, we may avoid talking about his future plans with him, we may evade his questions about his condition. Unwittingly, we have told him indirectly that he is dying. Patients who become aware that they are dying may not put this into words as they prefer to cope with the situation on their own. Some will never be aware that they are dying and it would be cruel to tell them if they do not question their increasing weakness, the progress of their illness or their prognosis. It should therefore never be a policy to tell everybody everything, but let each individual lead the way in what he wants to know and when.

Common Reactions to Dying

After a person has been told he is dying, it is important for the one who gave him that information not to leave him. He/she should stay and sit quietly ready to respond to the patient's reaction. There may be tears or initial disbelief and shock. He may say things such as, 'It can't be true'. 'The results of my tests have been mixed up with someone else's'. Denial is an understandable response to unwelcome news. It takes time for the person to absorb what the doctor or nurse has told him. The teller should therefore give the person time to react to the news in his own way. There may be immediate questions that he wants to ask concerning the length of time he has to live, whether or not his relatives know, and the likely course of the illness. The doctor or nurse should respond honestly to him and give him the information he seeks in a simple, kind and direct manner. He should be reassured that the staff are there to help and support him to the end.

Some patients will continue to deny that they are dying up to the time of their death. This may be a necessary defence mechanism for them and the only way that they can cope with the news. Their response must be respected. Nothing will be achieved by trying to force a person to acknowledge that he is dying. Other people, once they have taken in the fact that they are dying, will accept it but then other feelings of fear, loneliness, anger or depression may begin.

Fear

Patients who are dying often have various fears which can be allayed by the nurse when the patient puts his particular fear into words. Some are frightened that their pain will not be controlled. Today, we have at our disposal a wide range of analgesics, some of which are very strong (see Chapter 4) and it is rare for anyone to die in intractable pain. It is therefore possible for the nurse to reassure the patient that he will be given adequate pain killers to relieve the pain or at least make it bearable.

Another common fear is one of death itself as an unknown experience. No one is able to say what death is like, but the nurse's experience of death in other patients which is usually quiet and peaceful may give the dying person the comfort he seeks. The majority of people are unconscious at the moment of death, and telling the patient that he is likely to die in his sleep may reassure him. Actually seeing another patient die peacefully on the ward may reinforce the nurse's words.

Another fear of the dying is that they will lose control of themselves, physically and mentally. Loss of physical control may manifest itself in incontinence, generalised weakness or paralysis. Some patients find it difficult to accept their increasing dependence on others. The nurse's approach to their loss of physical control may help or hinder this acceptance. If she has a calm, kind manner and treats the patient with gentleness and respect he will find it easier to accept his loss of independence.

Some fear that they will lose their self-control towards the end. They fear that they may not have the courage or strength to endure dying, but will cry out against God and blame others. The likelihood of this happening is very rare and therefore the nurse can reassure the patient of this. At the same time patients who are dying are often emotionally labile and cry easily. The nurse should allow this as it is a natural outlet for fears and can ease mental suffering. The nurse can tell the patient that tears do help, especially if the dying person is a man.

Allied to the fear of the loss of physical and mental control is the feeling of helplessness which dying people may experience. They are powerless to stop the dying process and this can make them frightened and overwhelmed by a situation which they cannot avoid. For people who have always had a firm control over their lives this can be a frustrating and demoralising experience. Perhaps for the first time they find themselves in a situation where they are not in charge. Those around them, the medical and nursing staff, have some control over the dying process but they are not able to stop its inevitable end in death. The patient should be encouraged to control aspects of his care such as the timing of a wash or the choice of a drink. He should also be fully involved in decisions about changes in his drugs and treatment so that he can understand why they are being made as an indication that the situation is being controlled.

Other people fear losing their health and strength at this particular time in their lives. For example, a man who has just retired and has made many plans for his increased leisure time, suddenly sees all these hopes shattered when he discovers that he has a terminal illness. He needs time to adjust to this change in his life and to re-focus his plans on the more immediate future rather than long term arrangements. Here the family can help by encouraging him to set his sights on a more limited range which can be achieved. For example, they can plan a weekend away together rather than a long holiday abroad.

Little worries or fears may cause more outward anxieties than large ones. For example, one man may spend a lot of time and energy worrying about the functioning of his colostomy rather than the fact that he is dying. The nurse should be sympathetic and show understanding about the little worries so that in time, if the patient senses that she is concerned about small worries, he may confide in her about a great, deeply seated fear or worry.

Loneliness

Loneliness is a common feeling when anyone first learns that he is dying. It has been said that death is probably the loneliest experience that a human being has to face during his lifetime. He is surrounded by people who are not dying, such as nurses and his own family and friends. This can make him feel isolated. It is a policy in some hospitals for dying patients to be nursed in a sideroom away from other patients. This should be avoided unless the patient specifically requests to be on his own, or his symptoms are distressing to others, since the sideroom may increase his sense of loneliness and abandonment. Companionship of fellow patients in hospital and his family and friends at home can ease the feeling of isolation.

Nurses should make a point of going up to a patient and saying a few words to him at odd times during the day and not just when they have duties to carry out. Doctors also should be encouraged to include the dying patient on their ward rounds. Sometimes doctors avoid the terminally ill and go past the end of the bed as they do not know what to say. They may feel helpless because the patient is no longer responding to active treatment. In this situation the nurse can assist her medical colleague by suggesting questions for him to ask the patient such as 'Is the pain-killing medicine working effectively?' 'How is your appetite?' By guiding the doctor in this way he will not pass by the patient and increase his sense of isolation. He should ask, 'How are you?' looking at him and waiting for an answer. Closeness suggests warmth, and it is better to go to his side than to address him from the foot of the bed.

Relatives may also need help from the nurses about how to include the patient in day-to-day happenings at home, and to encourage hobbies and other pastimes. In hospital relatives should keep the patient in touch with what is going on in the outside world and include them in family news and decisions.

Anger

Anger is another common reaction when a person knows that he is dying. He may ask, 'Why has this happened to me? I have lived a good life.' Others, especially the young, see themselves with everything to live for — a career with good prospects, a loving wife or husband, perhaps a young family — and it is all being taken from them because they have an illness which is going to result in death. Naturally, they are very resentful. How does such anger and resentment reveal themselves? A patient may be very demanding about his nursing care. He gets impatient when care is not carried out on time or to his liking. Nothing is right. He criticises the nurses, the doctors, his treatment. He may argue with his family. This type of behaviour is difficult to deal with. The nurse should not respond by getting cross and impatient herself, but approach the patient calmly and politely however provoked she feels. All his requests should be met where possible. Given time and attention, and treated with patience and understanding, most patients eventually respond by being courteous and polite in return.

It may be necessary for the nurse to support the relatives when a patient is venting his anger on to them. She can try and explain his behaviour and that the family should not blame themselves. They should try to be patient themselves and he will eventually respond to their love and attention.

Depression

Depression is an understandable reaction to the knowledge that one is going to die. The dying patient grieves over his impending loss not only of his life but of his family, friends, a favourite pet, a stimulating job. Grief is a necessary preparation for a person's final separation from this world. The dying person should be allowed to express his sorrow at losing all he loves in whatever way is appropriate for him. For some, crying is of help, others find prayer a comfort, others want to talk. The nurse can help by providing a sympathetic hearing and privacy for the patient. She can tell the hospital chaplain or the patient's own minister and arrange for them to be alone in a quiet place. Some people find it helpful to reminisce about their lives. The nurse should not be tempted to cheer the patient up or ask the doctor to prescribe an antidepressant. Sorrow is a natural reaction to coming death, and the patient should be given the opportunity to express his sorrow, and hopefully through it achieve acceptance and peace.

There may be other causes of depression. The patient may feel guilty about some misdemeanour, real or imaginary, in the past, or wish to resolve a broken relationship. The nurse

can help by contacting the appropriate minister or
that the patient is able to make a confession, and be
The nurse may also be able to arrange for the e
relative to visit in order to achieve a reconciliation
him and the patient. This will lead to peace of mind for the
dying.

There may be feelings of shame if the patient is incontinent,
or there is an unpleasant odour from a fungating wound or
discharge. The nurse's attitude to these is important for the
patient; if she has a kind accepting approach and cares for the
patient with efficiency and gentleness this will restore his
self-esteem and confidence.

It is perhaps useful to point out that a dying person's moods
and attitudes are transient. He may be depressed one day and
optimistic and hopeful the next day. The nurse should therefore adapt her approach to the patient accordingly, sharing
his sorrow on one day and joking with him the next. A long
face and permanent air of gloom have no place when one is
nursing the dying. A quiet smile, a gentle touch on the shoulder can reassure the dying that they matter, and that they are
accepted for themselves with all their ups and downs and
different moods. The value and worth of each dying individual
must be recognised.

Acceptance

There are people who, given time, accept their approaching
death calmly and peacefully. They have worked through their
feelings of anger, questioning, depression and grief, and they
now wait patiently for the end. Such a calm acceptance can be
distressing for relatives as the patient may appear distant and
less talkative. He has reached the point where he is leaving
behind tiredness and sickness rather than life with all its
attendant attractions. What the dying man needs at this
time is the presence of his nearest and dearest, and the reassuring clasp of someone's hand rather than a lot of talking and
general bustle.

Some patients accept death early on in their illness because
their philosophy of life encompasses a belief that illness,
suffering and death are part of the human condition. Others
accept death because of their religious convictions. Their firm

belief in God helps them to cope with the fact that they are dying. Death is not seen as the end of life but a new beginning.

Patients who do accept their dying usually have an air of serenity about them and a quiet strength which carries them through all the ups and downs of their illness. However there may be times when they do feel anxious, frightened and doubtful of the future. The nurse can then intervene and reassure them and help them to regain their serenity. Even when people have accepted the fact that they are dying, they need to live until they die. It is therefore the nurse's responsibility to encourage whatever the dying person sees as living for him. It may be the smoke of a favourite pipe, the re-telling of a memorable occasion in his life, the smell of roses. Whenever possible the nurse should try and meet these requests.

Beliefs About Death

When someone is dying he may seek, for the first time, the meaning of life and death, and this inevitably involves philosophical and religious beliefs. A person's belief and outlook on life will influence the way in which he views death. How can the nurse help a patient who is trying to sort out his beliefs? She can listen carefully to his expressions of belief, and when the person has a religious faith she can ask his minister or priest to visit, with the patient's permission. It is important to bring the minister in early on in a person's illness rather than leaving it until the last few moments of life. This is in order for the minister to build up a trusting relationship with the patient and his family which can continue after death to support those left behind. Hinton (1971 *Dying*, Penguin) found that dying people with a firm religious faith or no faith at all are the most free from anxiety when they are dying. Tepid believers, who professed a faith but with no outward observance of it, were noticeably more anxious.

Dying patients with a religious belief should be given every opportunity to practise their faith in ways that are meaningful for them. The various practices and rituals associated with different religions are described in Chapter 1. The role of the nurse in providing spiritual comfort should not be undervalued as she or a colleague is with the patient twenty-four hours a day. Sometimes spiritual needs arise most strongly at night when it is quiet and the person has time to think about his beliefs. Usually the nurse is the only person available at night, although most ministers will gladly come if they are contacted. The night nurse can listen to the patient, and she may be able to help by reading a passage of scripture to him if this is acceptable.

Not all dying people feel the need for spiritual help, so it should not be forced upon them whatever the nurse's own religious faith may be. A person's belief or non-belief is his own affair and the nurse must accept this and only offer her assistance when she is asked.

Dying Person's Relationships with Others

When a person is dying his relationship with his family and friends may undergo changes. His role in society may alter because he is now ill and dying rather than well and healthy. A man who was a successful business man, enjoyed sport and was the head of his family now finds himself having to hand over his work to others to continue after his death. Because of weakness he has given up sport and his family are having to learn to manage without him. This results in a lowering of his self-esteem and he may express a wish to die sooner rather than later as he finds it difficult to accept his changed position at work and at home. Because he is trying to adjust to his change in role his behaviour may be very demanding and at times unreasonable. He may keep ringing his bell for trivial requests and complain about everything. The reason for such behaviour is that he is trying to retain some measure of independence and authority.

The nurse should respond to his behaviour by patiently acceding to his wishes where possible and showing him tolerance and kindness, no matter what she feels. This can be very difficult and it may be helpful to discuss the patient's behaviour with colleagues so that the burden is shared. It is important for the nurse to reassure the patient that he, as a person, still matters, and that he has an important role to play in teaching his family how to cope with finances and other affairs, and his business colleagues how necessary it is to give him some decisions to make and involve him in future plans even though he will not be there. In his nursing care the patient should be allowed to decide as much of it as possible so that he retains some independence.

There may be other people who seemingly were the weak ones in the family, but now that they are dying, find that they can be strong and help the family adjust to their coming death. In these circumstances the nurse may be needed as an emotional outlet for the patient after he has been comforting the family. This may mean accepting fears or giving a sympathetic ear to listen to the patient's outpourings. It is the nurse's responsibility to make sure that the patient is not over-burdened by the emotional demands of the family. She can do this by offering her support to the family and suggesting shorter visits for a few days if this seem appropriate.

In an intimate relationship like marriage the fact that one of the partners is dying may draw them closer together and they can share their joys and their sorrows. They learn to live one day at a time and make each day a memorable one in some way. Then, after death, the remaining partner will have precious memories to cherish. The nurse can assist in this by giving the couple opportunities to be alone together and expediting outings or other activities they wish to do together.

Conversely, if there have been trials and tribulations in a marriage they may be emphasised when one of the partners is dying. Both may feel guilty about the past but cannot be reconciled to each other. Sometimes a reconciliation does take place, but when it does not a tense atmosphere may exist between the two which may then spread to other members of the family. It may be too late to patch up an unhappy marriage at the stage when one of the partners is dying. The nurse can only offer support and understanding to both the dying and his partner.

In conclusion, the psychological care of the dying encompasses a wide range of emotions and feelings. It involves the patient himself, his family and friends and members of the caring team. The nurse's role is to provide an outlet for the various emotions and to give help and comfort whenever she can. To do this she will need the support of her colleagues as it can be very demanding on her own emotions and feelings.

However, it remains a great privilege to care for the dying, physically, psychologically and spiritually.

7

Care of the family

When most people die they leave behind relatives, friends and colleagues who will mourn their death but who will, with time, gradually learn to adjust to life without that particular person. There are a few people whose death will affect no-one except perhaps fleetingly those who have been acquainted with them in hospital or at home. This chapter is concerned mainly with families who lose a dearly loved member. It deals with relatives who have to adjust to a sudden and unexpected death in the family, and with those who have to come to terms with someone's death after a long and perhaps painful illness. There is a brief section about the family of a suicide victim.

When a family has to face the fact that a well-loved member of it is dying, they experience a variety of emotions. These emotions will depend on the depth of the relationship that each member has with the dying patient, the duration of the illness and the type of death. There are families in which all the relatives rally round and support each other and those outside the family, such as other patients and their relatives. Other families are small and closely knit and only become involved with their own dying relative. They also support each other but in a tighter circle.

When a family is told that a member is dying, they go through similar emotions to the dying patient himself when he is given the news. If the death is expected after a long or short illness the family has had some time to get used to the idea of losing a loved member. However, if the death is sudden there will have been no period of adjustment. If the death is due to suicide, again the family may be taken by surprise or they may possibly have been anticipating it. These three types of death will be considered separately as the emotions experienced by the family will be different for each.

The Family of a Patient whose Death is Unexpected

When a patient is brought into hospital in a serious condition following an accident or sudden onset of an illness, such as a stroke or heart attack, there has been no preparation in the family to face this situation. Usually they are summoned to the hospital by the police or by a telephone call, and they arrive in a state of shock. It is difficult for them to believe that, for example, the father and husband who left home fit and well is now dangerously ill. A nurse should be on the alert for them and conduct them to a quiet room away from the bustle of the casualty department or the intensive care unit. The doctor should see them and explain as gently as possible what has happened and how the patient is being treated. The family are given time to absorb the news and ask questions. Before they visit the patient they should be warned by the nurse about any equipment that is being used such as a respirator, and also if the person's face or body is disfigured.

In some cases the family may have to wait a long time before they can see the patient because he needs emergency care and surgery. Waiting can seem endless to relatives and the nurse can help by frequent short visits to them to keep them up-to-date with what is happening, to answer their questions if she can, and to meet their needs of rest and refreshment. When the family do see the patient, they may be shocked by his appearance and upset, especially if he is unconscious. They will probably have more questions to ask. It is essential that staff are as honest as possible about the patient's prognosis in order to give the family a chance to come to terms with his likely death. Sometimes the family are in a mild state of panic, and need guidance from the nurse about organising essential affairs, for example, getting the children collected from school.

A word should be said at this point concerning the approach to the family for permission to use some of the patient's organs for transplantation in the event of death. Before such an approach is made it is essential that the family understand the full extent of the patient's injuries and the likelihood of his death. There have been cases where the family were asked about transplantation before they realised how ill the patient was. The nurse who is in close contact with the relatives may be able to advise the doctor about how the family are reacting to the patient's condition, and also whether their religious belief condones or condemns the donation of organs. (Approaches about donation of organs from patients who survive longer and have life-support systems have been considered in Chapter 2.)

While the patient remains gravely ill, either in the ward or in the intensive care unit, the family need support from the nurses. They may be anxious about whether the patient is in pain or aware of what is going on around him if he is in a coma. The nurse needs to explain that he will be kept free of pain, and that he may be able to hear them, and tell him who is visiting. The family may worry about small attentions to detail, such as clean sheets, rather than the life-saving machinery. They may feel angry that the person is dying, and this may show itself in the form of demanding behaviour, or blaming the doctors for not doing all they can for the patient. They may also blame God or themselves for what has happened. The nurse should listen to any outbursts calmly and not be tempted to retaliate. Feelings of depression and sadness are common. These may manifest themselves in tears. Crying is a normal expression of grief. The nurse can help by encouraging relatives to cry and providing privacy for them. Sometimes reminiscing about the patient as he was can ease the death.

When death does occur, the family need a place to relax and express their grief. They may want to return and view the body when the various tubes, intravenous lines and other apparatus have been removed. Seeing the body often helps their acceptance of the death. The nurse's role immediately after death is fully described in Chapter 8.

The Family of a Suicide Victim

Death by suicide is an unexpected death although there may

have been some warning signs from the victim that he was thinking about suicide. The family of someone who commits suicide is in a particularly vulnerable position. The victim may have been very depressed, and talked about 'ending it all' but he was not taken seriously. He may have made a suicide attempt already. Conversely, he may have given no indication that he was going to commit suicide. Inevitably the family will feel guilty and ask themselves who was to blame. Sometimes the suicide victim kills himself either in such a way or in such a place which will give the most pain to other people. He may leave a note describing the circumstances or naming those responsible for his death. This can be very upsetting for those concerned.

The way in which a family reacts to the suicide of one of its members depends on the relationship between the victim and the various members of the family; the circumstances surrounding the suicide; and each member's previous experiences with death and suicide. Responses by individuals to the suicide of a loved one may vary from intense grief, to feelings of guilt and even to relief if the victim has been in severe mental or physical pain. A relative of someone who takes his own life may blame himself or herself for not discovering him sooner and perhaps preventing death by getting him to hospital. This is particularly the case with a child whose father or mother commits suicide. The child may be haunted by the fact that, if only he had come home earlier or run for help more quickly, the parent might still be alive. Sometimes other adults try to hide the fact that a parent's death was caused by suicide. This is usually a mistake as the child will eventually find out what happened and may be very distressed that he was not told the truth at the beginning.

How can the nurse help the family of someone who has committed suicide? As with other bereaved families, she can encourage them to talk about the one who has died. She can give them the opportunity to express their feelings and responses to the suicide. Relatives may need reassurance that they could not have prevented the individual from taking his own life. They will also require long-term support as they go through the normal process of mourning which is associated with bereavement. This support may be provided by a health visitor or a community psychiatric nurse if the latter was visiting the victim prior to his suicide. He may then continue to visit in order to help the family come to terms with what has happened.

The Family of a Patient who has a Chronic Terminal Illness

When a family first learns that a loved one has an illness which may ultimately result in death, such as liver failure, multiple sclerosis or cancer, again their initial reaction may be shock and disbelief. This feeling will probably not be as pronounced as the family whose relative is facing imminent death, but it does take them time to adjust. With some diseases a cure is possible, for example, many forms of cancer are now successfully treated, but with other illnesses the disease process continues until death ensues. The family has to learn to readjust itself to life with a person who is slowly dying of a sometimes very disabling condition. The special problems of the parents of a dying child are discussed in Chapter 11.

Having someone with a chronic illness in the home can put a strain on family relationships. The affected person may resent being dependent on others for some or all of his needs, and this may show itself in irritability and impatience. Often one family member takes the main burden of caring for the ill one, and this can become a great physical and mental strain. In these cases the support of the community nurse is vital. She can provide physical nursing care and can be an outlet for the frustrations of the patient. In some families there are enough family members for them all to rally round and share the care. However they will probably still need the expertise of the community nurse on methods of physical management and to provide moral support and encouragement.

When an individual is dying the family may wish to shield him from the true nature of his illness. This wish may be because they feel it would upset him too much to know, or because they could find it difficult to cope with their own emotions if he knew. It was explained in Chapter 6 that there is no hard and fast rule about how much a person should be told about his illness, when, and by whom. However, if the consensus of the staff is that he should be told, the family need an explanation of the reasons for this decision. It can be explained that it would be wrong to lie to the patient if he asked outright. Also he may want to know in order to put his affairs in order. It can soften the blow if it is pointed out that the patient realises he is getting weaker and probably has guessed the reason anyway. In circumstances where the family feel they are not going to be able to manage their own emotions if the patient knows, the nurse can reassure them that she and her colleagues will be there to help them. Usually when there is complete honesty between the dying person, his family and the staff, there is an atmosphere of warmth and trust.

During the course of chronic illness and particularly when the disease enters its final stages, the family has time to adjust themselves to life without that individual member. This has been termed 'anticipatory grieving'. It means that the family goes through the phases of mourning before the person dies. These phases are described in detail later (p. 82) but may be summarised as: an overwhelming sense of loss, deep sorrow, guilt, anger and depression. A few people successfully move through these phases and accept quietly the death of the loved one. It used to be thought that people who had done much of the 'grief work' before death had a shorter time of grieving afterwards. With some families this is certainly so, but others may go through all the normal phases of grieving again. What does this mean for the nurse? She may need to explain to relatives that it is usual and acceptable to grieve for someone before he or she dies. It is a very natural reaction when a person changes his personality as a result of his illness, or an elderly person becomes demented and no longer recognises her children and grandchildren. Because the patient may also be coming to terms with his death, he may be at a different stage of grieving than his family. The nurse can assist by explaining this to both the parties involved. It may happen that a person enters hospital for what is thought by all to be his last stay, but he recovers sufficiently to go home again. This situation can be very distressing, particularly if a wife has tried to prepare their children for his death and then father reappears at home. The role of the nurse is to try and understand and give support.

Many patients are able to die at home surrounded by family and friends and given support and help by the community nurses. The nursing care they require is discussed in Chapter

10. Other patients return to hospital or a hospice to die because they may not have relatives who can nurse them at home, or they may have distressing symptoms which need treatment, or the family may no longer be able to care for them for a variety of reasons. When a dying patient arrives in the ward, he and his family are kindly greeted and he is settled comfortably in bed or an armchair if he prefers. Any obvious distressing symptoms, such as pain, is dealt with immediately. It is helpful to talk to the family about how they have cared for the patient at home, as often they may have useful tips about the best way to turn the patient or give him his medicine. This information is recorded on the nursing care plan as an aid to the nurses.

The family may be feeling guilty because the patient has had to come into hospital. The nurse can reassure them that they have done their best, and she can encourage them to continue some aspects of the patient's care if they wish. Often there is a tendency in hospital to send relatives out of the ward when turning a patient or attending to his hygiene. When the family have been doing this at home themselves for weeks or months, they may wish to stay and help. This should be allowed provided that they are not over-taxing their own strength.

When relatives come to visit the dying patient, the nurse can show her care and concern for them by asking after them and how they are managing at home. There may be financial or other problems which the nurse can refer to the social worker. There may be behaviour difficulties with one of the children if a parent is dying. By building up a helpful relationship with the family before death, the nurse is able to assist them after death. Relatives always ask the nurse how the patient is. It is best to be honest with them if his condition is deteriorating, but to temper this with other personal information such as what the patient managed for lunch, or that he enjoyed a short trip out in the hospital grounds. The family often seek reassurance that their loved one is not suffering and it is usually possible to tell them that the medicine is keeping him free of pain.

Sometimes the strain that the family is under breaks through in the form of tears or an outburst of anger usually directed towards the staff over some detail of care. The nurse must understand that families do react emotionally in a variety of different ways to approaching death, and she therefore provides appropriate support. This may mean taking the family to a quiet place away from the public eye of the ward to cry, or listening patiently to their criticisms about the patient's care and endeavouring to correct it. Some families become over-tired with long daily visits to the patient, and may need advice from the nurse about taking the occasional day off. A few of the hospices have an official day off once a week for the visitors so that relatives can have a well-earned break and not feel guilty about it.

Towards the end of their life, many patients lapse into periods of unconsciousness. It is sometimes difficult for the family to decide who should stay with the patient. Usually one or two members emerge who are happy to remain at the bedside. Other relatives should be reassured that they have done all they can, and therefore it is right for them to go home and rest. One relative should be delegated to ring the ward periodically to see how the patient is, and then relay the information to the others. Those who stay with the patient are the nurse's responsibility and her duties towards them are described next.

Care of the Family after the Patient's Death

Once someone has died the nurse's responsibility for the care of his family does not cease but remains until such time as her support and help are no longer required. Although the hospital nurse usually has limited contact with the family after the patient's death, she needs to be aware of the help that her colleagues in the community can give to the bereaved. The health visitor or community nurse often provides the main means of support to families who have lost a loved one. She can offer them advice on the practical procedures which are necessary after a death, and give them an outlet to express their grief and to mourn.

When a patient actually dies, whether in hospital or at home, it is usually the nurse who has to convey the news to the family. The initial response to telling someone that a loved one has died is shock and disbelief. This will be particularly pronounced if the death was sudden and therefore unexpected, for example a fatal heart attack with no previous symptoms. If the patient has been terminally ill for several weeks or months his family will have had time to prepare for bereavement. However, the moment of death may still cause mild shock. If the relatives were not present at the death in hospital, it is important to tell them in privacy where they can show their grief. The sad news should be conveyed with honesty and sympathy.

There may be physical symptoms of distress such as waves of deep sighing, muscle weakness and choking sensations. There is a sense of unreality and numbness. The nurse's role at this time is to be with the family and let them express their feelings. Words from them, such as 'It can't be true', 'He isn't dead', should be listened to and not negated as they will slowly realise the truth of what has happened. A brief word from the nurse telling the family how sad she feels about what has happened may help, but often her presence comforts more than many words.

The relatives may need reassurance that the person did not die in pain or did not ask for them at the end if they were not there. Relatives who were not present at the death may wish to view the body. In the case of sudden death this may be necessary in order for them to realise that their loved one is dead. It is the nurse's responsibility to ensure that the dead person looks as respectable as possible. If he was the victim of a violent death, attempts should be made to wash away blood and dirt, and swathe the head in a covering if there is trauma to the brain. Some hospitals have a chapel of rest, where the body may be viewed in peaceful surroundings.

Emotional Responses to Bereavement

Losing a loved one is a very painful experience for most people. During the first few weeks after the death, the bereaved are often in a state of emotional shock. They feel numb, and although they can usually cope with the practical arrangements, the full impact of grief does not hit them until after the funeral. It is then that the process of grieving begins. Grief is the normal response to bereavement, and is necessary in order for the bereaved to come to terms with the loss of a loved one. It is a painful period of adjustment as the mourner learns to live without the mourned. If attempts are made by well meaning friends or others to try and curtail grief in the sufferer, or hurry him through the process, irreparable damage may be done to his mental state. Grief may be arrested at a certain point only to recur when another relative dies, but this time the reaction will be more overwhelming than before. It is therefore important for nurses to understand the normal mechanisms of grief.

Grieving for a loved one who has died is a time of intense sorrow and pain. It may take up to two or more years to resolve depending on the personality of the individual involved. A variety of feelings are experienced including an overwhelming sense of loss, guilt, anger, preoccupation with the image of the deceased, and identification with the dead person.

The sense of loss encompasses a wide range of subjects. When a member of a family dies he or she leaves a gap which has to be filled. The family must decide who is going to take on the various tasks of the dead person, such as paying the bills or getting in the coal. This can be very painful to decide. There are also continual reminders around the house of the dead person— his pipe on the mantelpiece, 'his' armchair in the sitting room, his clothes in the wardrobe. The daily routine is disrupted and can lead to feelings of lethargy and aimless activity. It can also mean that a place may be laid automatically for him at the table before the widow realises what she has done and consequently feels very upset.

If it is a child who has died the parents may want to have another of their own or to adopt a child to replace their loss. When one partner of the marriage dies and there are no children the remaining partner may be very lonely. Many of their social activities were participated in together and it may be difficult for a widow or widower to face such activities alone and without the support of her husband or his wife. The organisations such as *Cruse* for the widowed and their dependents may be able to help. When a homosexual relationship is divided by death, the one who is left behind is even more socially isolated than the widow or widower. It is hard for others to understand the feelings of the bereaved homosexual partner and there is very little support available for him or her as there is for the widowed.

Feelings of guilt may be experienced in a variety of circumstances. The mother of a child killed in a traffic accident may
blame herself for not teaching him road safety adequately.
The daughter of an elderly man who died in hospital may feel
guilty that she did not nurse him at home until the end, even
though he needed a lot of skilled nursing care. Some people
may feel that they contributed towards their loved one's death,
for example, the husband who died of a stroke after an argu-
ment with his wife. Others may blame themselves for not
recognising symptoms of a fatal disease earlier and urging the
person concerned to seek medical advice. Such feelings have
to be worked through by talking to others who will listen
sympathetically. Sometimes the doctor may need to reassure
the family that their action or lack of it did not contribute to
the death. The nurse may comfort the family that they did all
they could in caring for him either in hospital or at home. The
important thing is that the bereaved are allowed to talk freely
about their thoughts without being judged.

Anger may be expressed in several different ways. The
bereaved person may feel angry with the dead person for
dying and leaving him or her alone to cope. Although such
feelings pass, the person may feel horrified at himself for
thinking in that way towards the one he loved. Anger may
also be expressed towards the medical staff for not being able
to treat the person successfully or not diagnosing the disease
early enough. Irritation may be felt with the nursing staff for
what the bereaved person sees as acts of neglect when the
patient was dying. For example, the nurses may be accused of
not answering the buzzer quickly enough. After death the
bereaved person may dispute the articles of clothing or valuables that the deceased had with him in hospital. All these
things are manifestations of grief and must be accepted and
tolerated.

Some bereaved people seem preoccupied with the person
who has died. They have an idealised picture of the dead
person and will not tolerate any criticisms however mild.
They may have vivid dreams that the deceased is still alive or
they may hear his voice or even see him. This can be very
disconcerting, and the bereaved person may feel he is losing
his mind. However, he can be reassured that these things are
normal for someone who is mourning a loved one and will

pass in time. There is sometimes an element of identification with the dead person — taking over his interests or mannerisms, and in a few people showing symptoms of the illness from which he died. Tolerance is the key to cope with this as it usually rights itself in time.

The Widowed

Although everyone will suffer a bereavement at some time in his or her life, the widow or widower is in a particularly vulnerable position. He or she has lost their partner in life, their lover, confidant and friend. When a couple have been married for many years they have become completely used to living with another person. When one of them dies the other has to make great adjustments and has to learn to live on his or her own again. Practical aspects of life which have to be altered include cooking meals for one instead of two, if there is no-one else living at home, making decisions on one's own instead of consulting with the other partner, and sleeping alone for perhaps the first time since he or she was married. There is a tendency for the widow or widower not to eat proper nourishing meals as there is no incentive to prepare them any more. In such situations neighbours and friends can help by inviting the widow or widower to their home for meals occasionally, and accepting the widow's hospitality if she offers them a meal.

Holidays can prove another stumbling block for the widowed. Before bereavement the couple probably planned and discussed holidays for months before they went. The husband was there to organise booking the holidays, buying the tickets and handling the luggage. The wife prepared for the holiday by laundering the clothes, packing them and organising a meal for the journey. When one of them dies, the onus of making holiday arrangements falls on the widow or widower alone. To go away on one's own requires courage, and many may not be able to face an hotel alone. Going with a friend may be the answer, or a coach tour where one can get to know others during the journey. The widowed may be invited to join a son or daughter and their family on holiday. There are also some holidays specifically designed for single and widowed people.

Abnormal Reactions to Grief

Although it has been stressed before that grieving is a natural reaction to the loss of a love one, there are some people whose grief goes beyond the normal limits. Nurses who care for the bereaved need to be aware of these abnormal reactions so that they can advise on where to seek more skilled help from a trained counsellor or psychiatrist. Such abnormal reactions to grief are usually the result of exaggerated and/or prolonged symptoms of normal grief. They tend to occur when there has been a delay or postponement of grief at the time of death. For example, a man may lose his wife at a time of crisis at his work, and he is unable to grieve properly until the work situation is dealt with. A woman whose husband dies may have to put on a brave face for the sake of the children. Sometimes well-meaning friends can halt grieving by telling the bereaved to cheer up and 'pull themselves together'. If grief has to be put off for whatever reason, when the bereaved does mourn, his grief may become severe and prolonged. Even if grief is not postponed, some people who lose a close relative or friend through death may react abnormally.

How does the nurse recognise that someone who has been bereaved is grieving in an abnormal way? One observation she may make is that his behaviour changes. A previously quiet and serious person may become over-active, and filled with a sense of well-being rather than loss. An outgoing, cheerful individual may withdraw from society altogether and shun any form of social contact. Some people become completely devoid of any emotional expression whether of joy or sadness. Another sign of abnormal grief is that the deep sorrow which is often felt changes into severe depression with accompanying insomnia, self reproach and even a tendency to suicide. Someone else may completely deny that death has taken place. He talks as though the dead person was still there, and also acts in a similar manner, for example, preparing two meals instead of one. Although those who are grieving sometimes sense the deceased's presence and may even think that they hear his or her voice, with an abnormal reaction to grief there are signs of hallucinations and a loss of contact with reality. The affected individual seems unable to relate to the present situation and may wander about aimlessly. A few people then turn to alcohol as a solace.

The nurse has to use her powers of observation and her knowledge of normal grieving patterns in order to assess an abnormal reaction in the bereaved client. Her plan of action is usually to seek the advice of the client's general practitioner. He can then decide whether to refer the bereaved for specialised help. The earlier the symptoms of abnormal grief are detected the easier it is to help the person concerned. If the nurse is doubtful about someone's reaction to a loved one's death, it is safer to refer him for help than to leave him.

8

Final duties to the patient

The last few hours of someone's life can be a memorable experience for his relatives, other patients if he is in hospital, and the care-givers. It is the nurse's responsibility to make that memory as painless as possible by the care and support she gives to the dying patient and to those around him. For the dying person himself she needs to ensure his comfort physically, emotionally and spiritually, and to make the end of his life peaceful and dignified.

In hospital it is sometimes difficult to decide whether a dying patient should be nursed in the main ward or in a sideroom. A conscious patient may either welcome the companionship of his fellows or prefer the privacy of a single room. Some patients feel that if they are moved to a sideroom they are being pushed out and may feel rejected and isolated. Others, who perhaps do not know that they are dying, interpret the move out of the main ward as a definite sign that death is near; they become very anxious and frightened. When a patient becomes unconscious it is easier to move him, but it is difficult to tell how aware he is. He may sense that he is on his own and feel afraid but is unable to communicate this. Other patients may not want their companion taken away from them as they wish to watch with him as death approaches. Conversely, fellow patients may be upset at someone dying in their midst and would like him moved. There are also the relatives to consider as some may wish to grieve while others welcome the support of surrounding patients and their families. These are a few of the aspects for a nurse to consider when she tries to decide where a dying patient in hospital should be nursed.

Most people lapse into unconsciousness as the hour of death approaches, although there are a few who will be conscious to the end. It is important for everyone around the dying patient to remember that hearing is the last sense to go. Therefore a seemingly unresponsive patient may be able to hear what is going on by his bedside. The nurse should always explain any care she gives before doing it. She can reassure relatives that their words of comfort and affection may still be reaching their unconscious loved one. If the patient is known to be a Christian, reciting the twenty-third psalm may help him, and similarly other religious words or poetry may be of comfort to others. The minister, priest or rabbi of the dying patient should be informed that the end is in sight so that he can visit and offer spiritual comfort to the dying and his family. (For details of the various religious practices see Chapter 1.) When a Roman Catholic receives the Blessing of the Sick this is noted in the records as it is an important rite for him to have before death. It is necessary for other nurses to know that he has had it so that they do not contact the priest for it again.

It is usually obvious to most experienced nurses when terminally ill patients have entered the last phase of life. Breathing changes in character and there may be pauses between respirations. Unless the patient shows signs of increasing dyspnoea, oxygen can be turned off and the mask removed so that his face can be clearly seen. If his breathing becomes noisy, the so-called 'death rattle', this is usually due to secretions collecting in the air passages which cannot be coughed up as the patient is too weak. Sometimes gentle suction at the back of the throat may clear it, but often the fluid is too far down in the bronchi for a suction catheter to reach. Repositioning the patient and lifting his jaw upwards sometimes eases the breathing. If not intramuscular atropine sulphate 0.6–1.2 mg or hyoscine 0.4–0.6 mg can be given to dry up the secretions. Relatives will need reassurance that the patient is not aware of his noisy breathing. Other patients may also be upset by the sound and require a kind explanation from the nurse.

The colour may drain from the dying patient's face and his

cheeks may sink in, giving him a rather haggard appearance which can be distressing for his family. He may be drenched in cold perspiration as his peripheral circulation fails, and yet be throwing off the blankets as his internal temperature is hot. He will feel cold to the touch and therefore his relatives may worry that he is not warm enough. Again a simple explanation by the nurse will help. Light bedclothes held off his legs by a bed-cradle and sponging away the perspiration will keep him comfortable. This may be a task that his family would like to do. A full blanket bath is usually no longer necessary, but a refreshing hands-and-face wash and hair tidying will suffice. Most dying patients are more comfortable on their side, well supported by pillows. Regular turning and repositioning is essential and keeping the lips moistened with sips of water and/or soft paraffin ointment.

If the patient has been receiving regular analgesia by mouth it is necessary to continue it when he is no longer able to swallow. Usually half the dose of analgesic given by mouth is sufficient administered intramuscularly. However the nurse should monitor the patient's condition carefully in case a higher dose is required. If the patient is restless, moving around in the bed and throwing off the bedclothes, although seemingly unconscious, some type of sedation may be required. It is advisable to check first that the patient is not suffering from retention of urine when passage of a catheter may relieve his restlessness. Otherwise, an injection of intramuscular diazepam 10 mg or chlorpromazine 25–50 mg may be given to sedate the patient and to comfort the relatives as well as himself.

The nurse should always bear in mind that the atmosphere created around the dying patient will remain with relatives, friends, other patients and junior nurses for a long time. From a physical point of view the patient should look well cared for with his hair combed, the face shaved if he is a man, and the sheets and pillowcases spotlessly clean. Apparatus close to the bed, such as suction machine, should be removed unless it is likely to be required, so that the family can actually reach and touch their loved one. There are people who are frightened of touching someone who is dying, and the nurse may need to encourage the relatives to hold his hand, stroke his cheek or do whatever seems natural to them. The dying patient should be peaceful and surrounded by tender loving care and concern. Loud conversation and laughter is out of place near the bedside of a person who is dying, but a warm smile can help not only the patient but his family and friends as well.

It is a privilege for a nurse to be present at the end of someone's life as it is to be there at a birth. Sometimes death comes almost imperceptibly, and it is hard to tell at exactly what point in time the patient died. On other occasions the actual death is more obvious as the noisy breathing stops or restlessness ceases. The doctor is asked to come and certify the death.

Once death has occurred the nurse's duty is to the relatives. She needs to tell them that their loved one has now died. She may say 'He has gone', or 'He is at peace now', or simply 'He has died'. If the family are not present at the death the nurse will have to contact them at home. Unless specifically asked to telephone at night, the nurse should inform the relatives in the morning if a patient dies during the early hours. It is also helpful for the nurse to know if there will be anyone with the relative when she telephones him. If the next-of-kin is elderly, it may be kinder to inform a younger member of the family. If at all possible, asking the police to tell a family of the death of a loved one should be avoided as it can be a shock to see a policeman standing at the front door.

Relatives who are present at the moment of death may be left alone with the body for a few minutes or the nurse may stay with them while they collect their thoughts. Some people like to kiss the body and stroke the face or hand. Others may throw themselves on the body either as an attempt to revive the corpse or as a final farewell gesture. Such outbursts of emotion should be tolerated as they are ways of helping the bereaved to come to terms with what has happened. It is their way of saying goodbye to a loved one. After a short while the family are usually ready to move away from the bedside. The nurse can escort them to a room away from the public eye where they can express their grief in private. Sometimes the nurse may need to indicate to the relatives that it is time to leave the bedside; she can either do this by words or by putting an arm round them and leading them away.

The family's initial response to the death varies. Some

members may cry openly while others remain silent. They may wish to reminisce about the person who has died and the nurse can be a sympathetic listener. She can also provide the facilities for one of the relatives to tell the news of the death to other members of the family, or she can offer to do this for them if they are very upset. A cup of tea is usually welcome. They may wish to speak to the doctor or to see the chaplain and the nurse can arrange this. After a period of time when the relatives feel composed, the nurse gives them the information about when to return to collect the death certificate, as described in Chapter 10. She then escorts them to the door of the ward or to the hospital entrance to see them on their way home. She can arrange for a taxi to take them home if necessary.

In a hospital or nursing home the other patients will probably realise that someone has died, but occasionally it may be necessary for the nurse to explain, especially if the death was unexpected. Patients should not be told that he has been moved to another ward. They are often fully aware of the death and it is a false assumption by the nurse that it will upset them too much to know the truth. Some of the patients may have become friends with the one who has died and they need the opportunity to grieve. A reassuring word from the nurse or a comforting hand to clasp is often enough to help them. Sometimes a brief explanation may be required for a patient with a similar condition who may be frightened of dying in the same way.

When junior and inexperienced nurses are involved in the care of the dying they may also be distressed when death comes. They need support from the senior nurse especially if the end has been upsetting; for example, a massive haemmorhage resulting in the death of the patient. Young nurses should never be made to feel ashamed if they shed a few tears for the dead. They should be reassured that this is a natural response to what has happened. It also indicates to the relatives that the nurses do really care about their patients. Clearly copious weeping is inappropriate and will not help the nurse or the relatives, so some control should be exercised. A nurse who is upset may benefit from taking a short tea or coffee break to compose herself or she may be better sent off to care for another patient. This depends on the individual nurse.

The final service that the nurse renders to her patient is that of last offices or laying out. In years gone by this used to be done by a senior member of the patient's family, but now it falls to the lot of the nurse and undertaker. There are a few hospitals today that have abolished full last offices. They feel it is more appropriate for nurses to spend their time with the living, and that other patients dislike a dead body in the ward for any length of time. In these hospitals the patient is straightened, and tubes or apparatus are removed and then the body is taken to the mortuary usually within half an hour of the death being certified by the doctor.

However, in most hospitals and nursing homes the nurses feel that laying out the body is the last service they can give to their patient. It helps them to come to terms with the death and enables them to prepare the body for its final resting place.

When death has been confirmed by the doctor the patient is laid flat on his back with no pillows. The eyes are closed, but if they stay open, two wet swabs are placed on the lids. Any tubes are removed, such as a urinary catheter, intravenous infusion or nasogastric tube. Drainage tubes are not taken out until later. Traction is dismantled and plaster casts cut off. Any urine remaining in the bladder is expelled into a kidney dish by applying pressure just above the pubic bone. If dentures were worn they are replaced and a pillow placed under the chin to prevent the jaw dropping and the mouth falling open. All clothes are removed, the limbs straightened and arms placed either side of the body. The body is covered with a clean sheet. All equipment is taken away and the bedside locker cleared except for a small vase of flowers or a cross.

If the dead patient is Jewish the nurse does only the minimum amount of preparation of the body. She puts on disposable gloves, closes the eyes, ties up the jaw and puts the arms straight by the sides of the body. Any tubes are removed and the incisions plugged with gauze and strapping. The body is then wrapped in a plain sheet and taken by the porters to the mortuary or other special room for Jewish dead. The body is then attended by members of the Jewish Burial Society.

With other patients it is customary to leave the body for one hour before returning to complete last offices. All necessary equipment should be collected beforehand on a trolley so that the nurses do not have to leave the bedside once they have started the procedure. Two nurses are usually required to facilitate turning. However, in the patient's own home the nurse may have to do last offices on her own.

In hospital if the second nurse is doing last offices for the first time, the senior nurse should remember this and act accordingly. Handling the dead for the first time may be viewed with apprehension by a nurse. Her senior explains that he will probably not feel cold as sufficient time for cooling after death has not elapsed. She points out that the limbs will flop as there is no life to support them, and that there may be a sighing sound when the body is moved. This is caused by the remaining air being expired from the lungs. If last offices are performed at night there should be adequate light so that the junior nurse is not made uneasy. Whenever last offices is performed it should be done with dignity and discretion.

The following equipment is used:

Bowl of warm water
Patient's toilet requisites
Towel
Wool and one pair of sinus forceps for packing the orifices if necessary
2 wool pads
Wide open-wove bandage
Dressing cut to size and waterproof strapping, if required for wounds and drainage sites
Shroud
Clean top sheet and drawsheet

The patient is washed and when the back is done, the anal canal is usually packed with a small piece of wool to prevent leakage. At the same time a clean drawsheet is placed beneath the body if necessary. A male patient is shaved. The hair is combed and arranged neatly. Finger nails and toe nails are trimmed if necessary. Any wounds are covered with a dressing and sealed with waterproof strapping. Sometimes there may be profuse drainage from a wound. Positioning the patient in such a way so as to encourage the secretions to drain out may help. Occasionally suction of the cavity may be performed to prevent seepage through the dressing. Final packing with a gauze roll held in place with waterproof strapping is done. Sutures are left *in situ*. A stoma is covered with a clean drainage bag. Any drainage tubes are removed and the site occluded with a waterproof dressing.

The nurses check that the body is correctly labelled with the patient's name, age, hospital number, religion and ward on a name band round his wrist. Some hospitals also have an identity band round one ankle to make it easier to identify in the mortuary. A shroud is then put on which fastens at the neck and wrists. Sometimes a wool pad is tucked inside the collar encircling the neck and improving the appearance. The ankles are fastened together using an open-wove bandage in a figure of 8 and a wool pad placed between the two malleoli. In some hospitals the whole body is wrapped up in a sheet while others leave a clean sheet draped over the body. The equipment is taken away and the porters are asked to remove the body. If the patient has a notifiable disease, such as viral hepatitis or tuberculosis, this information is passed on to the porters and the mortician.

It is customary to screen off the other patients' beds so that they do not see the arrival of the stretcher and the removal of the body. The property is listed and any valuables collected and signed for by the relatives. If a wedding ring or other jewellery is left on the body this should be recorded by two witnesses. The bed and locker are then washed and the bed made up with fresh linen. The nurse returns to her other patients.

9

Support for staff

After eight weeks in the School of Nursing, the learner nurse finds herself working full time with sick people, some of whom may be dying. As her training progresses she will meet terminally ill patients in a variety of situations; the elderly woman passing quietly away in a long-stay geriatric ward; the young man dying from multiple injuries in the intensive care unit after a motor cycle accident; a middle-aged man in a medical ward suffering from cardiac arrest; or a child dying from leukaemia. The way in which the junior nurse deals not only with these events, but with her own emotional reactions to them depends a great deal on how the senior staff react to them.

All nurses concerned with the care of a dying patient and his family should be fully informed of all relevant circumstances. They should be told whether the patient knows he is dying, and whether the family are fully aware of the diagnosis and likely outcome. Lay people attach meanings to some medical terms which are rather different from the technical ones. 'Cyst' and 'ulcer' are thought of as neutral words with no especially dire implications. 'Growth' and 'tumour' are serious words to them and imply malignancy. People who speak of their relative having an ulcer in the stomach may not be aware that it is a carcinoma.

Nurses must understand why active treatment (for instance, chemotherapy) is being withdrawn, and it should be made clear whether resuscitation is to be attempted or not in the event of cardiac or respiratory arrest. Many nurses encountering these problems for the first time ask themselves questions about the ethics involved, and these should be fully and sympathetically discussed and not brushed aside. Problems are more numerous today than they ever were because we have more mechanical ways of prolonging life than we used to have.

The chaplain of the denomination to which the student belongs may help to clear doubts and explain purposes.

The lady whose illness is described here had a series of heart attacks. It was decided that attempts to revive her, if she had another one, would not be in her best interests, in view of her extensive medical disease.

> One night at the beginning of December Mrs F. woke up fighting for breath and with severe chest pain. She woke her husband who called their general practitioner. He visited and made a provisional diagnosis of myocardial infarction. The doctor arranged her admission to a local hospital via the Emergency Bed Service. She was collected at home by ambulance and admitted to an acute medical ward with facilities for cardiac monitoring. In the ward the houseman examined her briefly and ordered intramuscular diamorphine 2.5 mg to be given immediately. This eased her pain considerably. The nurses made her comfortable in bed and attached leads to her chest wall, so that her heart could be monitored. Her husband, who had accompanied her to hospital, was then allowed in to see her after the cardiac monitoring had been explained to him. He was very relieved to see his wife relaxing in bed and no longer in pain. The nurse arranged for a taxi to take Mr F. home as it was too early for public transport to have started. Mrs F. was settled for the rest of the night with a cup of tea.
>
> During the next few days the nurses were able to learn more about Mrs F. She was 68 years old and her marriage to Mr F. was her second one. They were a devoted couple who had one daughter of their own, one adopted daughter and two daughters by Mrs F's previous marriage. All four visited Mrs F. regularly in hospital and laundered her pretty nightdresses and bedjackets for her.
>
> Mrs F. was no stranger to hospital. She had had chronic bronchitis for many years which necessitated treatment in hospital for chest infections in most winters. She often became short of breath when doing housework and found that she slept better sitting upright in bed. Her blood pressure was found to

be rather high. Two years ago she had had a stroke which had resulted in some left-sided weakness. Her grip was not strong in her left hand and she walked with a slight limp. She had a fair appetite and a tendency to constipation. Her usual medication included Navidrex K and Methyldopa for her blood pressure, Aminophylline Slow Release for her breathing and a long-term antibiotic, Oxytetracylcine, to prevent recurrent chest infections.

Mrs F. was a frail thin lady and was therefore nursed on a sheepskin from admission to prevent pressure sores. Due to her shortness of breath she found it difficult to lie on her side, but occasionally she managed this for a few minutes to relieve the pressure on her sacrum. She was an anxious lady who became very agitated when her breathing was bad. Sometimes her breathlessness was relieved by humidified oxygen via a 28% Ventimask. On other occasions the presence of her husband or a nurse to hold her hand and stay with her helped her to relax.

Mrs F's condition gradually improved after a few days in hospital with physiotherapy, drugs and careful nursing. She enjoyed sitting out of bed in an upright chair and would read the local newspaper or listen to the radio. She found chatting to other patients made her breathless after a short time. Her appetite improved a little when she was offered small portions at mealtimes, and strawberry-flavoured milk drinks in-between meals. She had a daily bowel action with the help of Dorbanex 10 ml at night. She had some difficulty in sleeping, but brandy in warm milk to settle her at night did help.

Ten days after admission to hospital Mrs F. began to deteriorate again. Her breathing became worse, she developed atrial fibrillation and ankle oedemia. The medical registrar diagnosed heart failure and prescribed an increased dose of diuretic and digoxin. At this stage the medical staff decided not to resuscitate Mrs F. if she had a cardiac or respiratory arrest. She had already had a severe myocardial infarct, and with her chronic lung condition her prognosis was poor. The registrar explained the situation fully to Mr F. and his daughters. The doctor then wrote in the medical notes and on the nurses' record that Mrs F. was not to be resuscitated. The ward sister made sure that all the nurses understood the reasoning behind this action. Mrs F. did not ask outright whether she would get better or not, but she was anxious about the chest pain returning. She was reassured by the medical and nursing staff that she could be given tablets or injections to stop the pain if it recurred.

Despite feeling very weak and breathless Mrs F. enjoyed Christmas Day and her husband had dinner with her on the ward. In the afternoon two of her daughters visited with one grandson. On Boxing Day Mrs F. complained of chest pain again. She was given two dihydrocodeine tablets but they did not help. The doctor then prescribed intramuscular diamorphone 2.5 mg which did alleviate the pain. The following day Mrs F's breathing was even more laboured and she lapsed into unconsciousness. Her husband stayed with her all day and into the night. He could occasionally be seen wiping tears from his eyes and would sometimes tell the nurses how kind and good she was. They listened sympathetically and made sure he was offered meals and cups of tea at intervals.

Mrs F. died peacefully at three o'clock in the morning with her husband holding her hand. Night sister comforted him and then he was left alone with his wife for a short while at his request. Night sister led him to the visitors' rest room where he had a cup of tea and managed to sleep until seven o'clock in the morning. Night sister arranged for one of his daughters to come and collect him.

When active treatment, such as radiotherapy or chemotherapy is stopped, or an operation is ruled out, it must not be thought that all treatment has been abandoned. A different course of treatment is to be used, in which the comfort and care of the dying patient is all-important, and in which the nurse has a major role.

Caring in the intensive care unit for a dying patient who is a potential donor of organs for transplantation involves inevitably conflict of emotions. The criteria for the diagnosis of death are described in Chapter 2. The nurse learns to do everything she can for her patient during his life, and to accept that he has died when these criteria are fulfilled. The switching off of a ventilator is not an act that causes death, but a recognition that death has already taken place. The nurse, like the family, may be able to feel glad that the death may mean life to someone else.

The caring team includes everyone from the consultant to the junior nurse, and all of these must be kept fully informed about the dying patient and his family. This depends on good relations and an effective means of communication between members. Many hospices have regular multidisciplinary meetings to discuss their patients and exchange information about them. This is also an opportunity for individual members to voice their own particular opinions and feelings, and if relations are good these feelings can be received, discussed and valued by the group.

A rather smaller proportion of patients, however, die in hospices than elsewhere. In hospitals, pressures of work and shortage of time may make such multidisciplinary meetings difficult and the gap between consultants and junior nurses may be inhibiting to real communication. The fact that communication is difficult should not make us relax efforts to maintain it. The ward sister provides liaison between the medical and nursing staff. She explains the situation about the patient and his family and offers guidance on how to answer possible questions that the patient or his relatives may ask.

A wide range of emotions is experienced by those who care for the dying. It is a normal reaction to grieve for those who die, and nurses have to learn how to recognise these feelings, and also how to control them for the sake of others. It is to be expected that nurses will become attached to some of their terminally ill patients, for a variety of reasons. They may relate to a young man or woman of their own age, or similar interests, who has malignant disease. A middle-aged patient may remind her of her father or mother, and this may intensify her emotional reactions. Nurses in many ways therefore relate to dying patients, and it is natural for them to grieve when one of them dies. It is perhaps more acceptable nowadays for a young nurse to express such grief. Although the trained nurse should help a junior to control an emotional outburst in the interests of her other patients, as well as herself, a comforting touch and a sympathetic word will give support.

There are special circumstances about some deaths which may cause more distress than usual among the staff. For example, death on Christmas Day causes conflict of emotions. Nurses are trying to help patients have a happy day, while sorrowing over the death of one of them. This is a time when a sideroom is a boon to relatives and staff, providing the patient agrees that he will find more peace away from the festivities, and relatives will appreciate not having to deal with the incongruity of festival and the approach of death. It is also obviously easier to deal with the formalities associated with dying if this does not occur in the general ward.

Many nurses start their training with no experience of death. It is therefore important that their introduction to death is handled tactfully and sympathetically. Seeing a dead person for the first time is an event which many view with confused feelings and apprehension. Some are really frightened about how they will feel when confronted with the finality of death, and if they will manage to control their reaction. When a death occurs on the ward the junior nurse should be given the opportunity to see the body. This can either be done with the dead patient in the position in which he died, usually resting on his side, or after he has been laid flat. The junior nurse should be accompanied by an experienced nurse and warned what to expect, e.g. the colour of the skin which may be very pale, tinged with blue, or have a mottled appearance. If she wishes she should be encouraged to touch the body. Afterwards she returns to the service of her other patients. It is a good idea to give her something specific to do for one of the other patients in order to stop her dwelling unduly on what she has just seen.

It may not be possible to protect a junior nurse from witnessing a disturbing death, e.g. from haemorrhage or respiratory obstruction, but her more senior colleague should offer some words of comfort and reassurance.

The performance of last offices is a procedure which is usually taught to nurses during their Introductory Course in the School of Nursing. At this stage most nurses regard it as a theoretical task and find it difficult to imagine putting it into practice. When a patient dies, last offices are sometimes regarded with apprehension by learner nurses mainly because of a fear of the unknown. They ask themselves questions such as 'What will the body feel and look like?' 'How will I react to laying out someone for the first time?' It is therefore important that a nurse's first experience of carrying out last offices is done with a qualified nurse or senior learner who is sympathetic and understanding about the nurse's fears.

The senior nurse should explain the procedure fully and warn the nurse what to expect, as described in Chapter 8 in the account of last offices. A sense of decorum is necessary during last offices to preserve a sense of dignity to the dead patient. The body should be handled reverently as if the individual was still alive. A disturbing first experience with last offices, either because the junior nurse is not given sufficient support by her senior colleague, or because the occasion is treated with indifference, can leave a long lasting effect on the nurse concerned. She may dread her next experience of dealing with a patient after he has died or she may become hardened herself. This in turn may lead to an unhelpful attitude to junior nurses when she is qualified.

When death happens unexpectedly, perhaps as a result of cardiac arrest when resuscitation was unsuccessful, the whole caring team may feel despondent. They ask each other if there was anything else they could have done to prevent it happening. Doctors may blame themselves for not doing more investigations. Nurses may question whether extra observation and vigilance on their part could have alerted them to the possibility of a cardiac arrest. It is important to allow these thoughts to be expressed, and then to accept that the team have done their best, but death could not be avoided. Occasionally one part of the team may be blamed, e.g. a piece of necessary equipment might not be working properly. Such recriminations are pointless at this stage. It is worth reminding each other sometimes that if the patient had not been in hospital when he collapsed it is likely he would have died anyway.

Those who come into contact with dying patients must learn to come to terms with death. This is not easy especially where children and young adults are dying of incurable disease. Voicing one's feelings with others may help, and although the ward sister should not encourage prolonged introspective discussions, some ventilation of emotions at report time may be of assistance to the nurses and may help those who are finding death difficult to cope with. Other nurses will turn to their friends or families for support. Nurses need to have the ability to react normally to grief when a patient dies, but with adequate restraint for the sake of other staff and patients.

To whom do the trained staff turn when they are particularly upset about a death? Most hospices provide a comfortable staff common room where nurses can retreat after a distressing death. The staff who are outside the immediate patient situation, e.g. the matron or chaplain, may be able to offer a few kind words of understanding. A short break away from the ward can give an essential breathing space and help the nurse to compose herself. Nurse managers should be alert to the needs of their staff. When there has been a particularly upsetting death on a ward, or in a house, or a run of deaths, senior nurses must watch for signs of tiredness, irritability, false cheerfulness or depression in their junior colleagues, and given them an opportunity to express their feelings in privacy. Nurses in the community are usually more isolated than their hospital peers. Informal meetings where difficult cases, including dying patients, can be discussed may be helpful. An understanding nursing officer who knows her district can be invaluable in giving support.

There are wards where there is an almost constant presence of death. Specialities, such as oncology and radiotherapy, invariably have patients who reach a terminal stage of their illness. They return to the ward for the last time where they have received active treatment in the past but are now dying. Permanent staff who work in these areas need to come to terms with malignant disease and death in order to remain sensitive to the requirements of their patients, and be able to accept death when it comes. Senior staff must also be mindful of the feelings of nurses seconded to the ward during training, and perhaps meeting terminal illness and death for the first time. Patients dying of malignant disease can look very distressing— they are often emaciated, sometimes jaundiced or oedematous. On the other hand, many cancer patients and their families face death with courage and learn to live a day at a time. Learner nurses can really benefit from experience with these patients if they are given adequate support, help and explanation by the trained staff.

It is not only the nurses who have to learn to cope with death. Doctors also find it difficult because they often feel a sense of failure when a patient dies. Deciding that a patient has reached the irreversible stage of his illness and can only be given palliative treatment is sometimes hard for a doctor to come to terms with. Some doctors react by spending the briefest possible time with dying patients, and ignoring his relatives, because they do not know what to say. The inclusion of more formal instruction for medical students on techniques of communication, and of attitudes to all patients and their relatives would be helpful. It is also possible for experienced ward sisters to guide young doctors in their role. It should not be thought by doctors that their sole function is to cure; when they are asked to give comfort or relieve symptoms in the incurable, they are using real medical and personal art. The doctor who passes a dying patient and his family is missing an opportunity of showing his real skill. He should stop by every patient's bedside, not at the end of the bed, feel his pulse, look at him, ask how he feels and listen to the answer. Relatives may ask, 'Can't you do anything for him, doctor?' and he should ask 'What do you think bothers him most?', and the answer may be pain, sleeplessness, lack of appetite, depression, any one of a variety of symptoms which the doctor can do something to help. He should also ask the relatives how they are. Good communication between doctors and nurses will ensure that all symptoms that can be treated are treated, and that they will agree when active treatment designed to effect a cure is no longer desirable. It does not make for good relations if nurses feel either that treatment has been abandoned too early, or carried on when it was a useless stress to patient and relatives.

Nurses are not of course the only staff who may need support over death. Domestic staff and ward clerks offer a different kind of service, but one which is vital to ward work. They may know some patients and their relatives well, and have shared their hopes and fears. The staff nurse or sister should speak to them about the death and allow them to express their feelings. Sometimes it may seem appropriate for them to see the patient after death, or to speak with the relatives.

Long Service Strains

There are many situations in which, from the nature of the work, death occurs often, and of course this invariably happens in hospices. Nurses must not expect that everyone will be able to undertake such work for an indefinite period, nor should they feel any sense of failure if they have to give it up. The average length of stay of a patient in a hospice is about six weeks, and the nurse must constantly bear in mind that her function is to give comfort, not to cure.

The early hospices were all-religious foundations, and the nuns who did the work expected to do so for life. They were united in a common religious belief that gave them a view of life and death in which they found support. Later they were joined by nurses of all religions, and of none, and the problems of these people were somewhat different.

The pace of work in a hospice is not fast, and in general the work is demanding because of the mental tension involved rather than the physical strain. Nurses find they must support and comfort patients and relatives, when sometimes they feel in need of comfort and support themselves. They are not confident of being able to answer questions like, 'Why does God allow suffering?' This kind of misgiving is just as common among Christians as it is among those who do not have a belief in God. It is only through thinking out their position, talking to colleagues, and listening to seniors dealing with such situations that they come to realise that people are not asking for a deeply-reasoned theological reply. Often they are not expecting any answer as such, but expressing pain and hoping for comforting words. We can tell them we feel for them, that it is hard to understand, that they must keep up their spirits in order to sustain the patient. Those of us who believe that there is this kind of God who 'allows' suffering, must also believe that He gives us the power to relieve suffering, and that we must strive to increase our knowledge and abilities to that end.

Nurses passing through this anxious, puzzled phase must be assured by their seniors that it can be worked through, and that those assailed by such anxieties often prove to be the sensitive, insightful people who have most to give. They should be encouraged to go out into the outside world, where there is so much marvellous life, in their off duty, and to seek to meet their friends, especially those with different work.

Later on a different kind of unhappiness may arise. Nurses may feel drained, depressed, indifferent and unable to give the kind of service that once was possible. Nuns too feel this kind of loss, and the nursing orders have many years of experience in dealing with it, and finding ways of relieving it with changes of post, of responsibility, and with holidays.

Nurses must not feel guilt if they find they can no longer carry on with work solely among the dying. While some have a lifelong dedication to this work, many more find there is a time to change. Many spend time in hospices in order to learn the expertise that they offer, and to use it when necessary in their own field, in the community or in hospitals.

10

Dying at home

The community nurse involved in the care of someone dying at home must have the clinical expertise of her colleagues in a hospice, but needs other qualities and knowledge in addition. She assesses the needs of the family as well as the patient, sets nursing goals for the caring group to achieve, and delivers or helps with the care.

Beyond this, the community nurse should show intuitive sympathy in noticing needs, and imagination in filling them. She must have the ability to teach the family, and to inspire them with confidence in their role. She must cooperate with the general practitioner and the social worker. She must have a good knowledge of the resources available to help the family, and see that they use these.

One of the great advantages of the patient being cared for at home in his final illness is the range of activity and choice of surroundings even in a small house. Someone dying in a hospital must, if he is bedfast, be in a room alone or in a ward with many others around. If he can get up, he may sit in a chair by his bed, or in a day room with the television on.

At home, patient and family and nurse can consider convenience of care and the patient's changing wishes and needs. It may be that he would like, while still retaining some power, to spend his day in the living room, where he can be with his loved ones, and look at his books or be involved with hobbies. A bed can be put up in the sitting room, or a settee arranged with rugs and pillows so that he can lie down during the day. A downstairs lavatory or a commode is convenient. Light people can be carried upstairs to bed. If the patient prefers quiet and seclusion, he can be nursed in his own bedroom, and his visitors can be regulated according to his wishes.

Nursing Care

Once the nurse has examined her patient, spoken with the family and seen the resources available in the home, she agrees with the family on the objectives to be reached. These are formulated in a way the family can understand; the nurse says 'This is what we're going to do'. While needs will vary greatly, they always include the following.

1. *Maintaining Personal Cleanliness and Freshness*

While it is still possible, the patient may be helped into a bath or given a shower. If this is not possible, the nurse gets the help of a relative in giving a bed bath, and probably can soon relinquish this task. She should however, from time-to-time assist with it; it gives her an opportunity to inspect the pressure areas, and to have time to talk and listen to the patient and the family.

2. *Preventing Pressure Sores*

These appear to be less common in people being nursed in their own beds than in those admitted to hospital. The reason for this is far from clear. There are, of course, more seriously ill people in hospital than there are at home, and the idea is supported more by general belief than by statistical proof. It is widely held by people who are nursing a chronically ill person at home that if he goes to hospital for any reason, he will get a pressure sore.

Appliances may be lent for home care; ripple mattresses, blocks to raise the height of the bed for convenience in nursing, sheepskins and cradles are examples. The community nurse will teach the relatives to use these, and also the best ways of lifting patients without straining the back.

3. *Obtaining a regular bowel action*

Prevention of constipation is just as important in the home as elsewhere. Relatives often say, 'He's taking so little, we can't expect a bowel action', but the importance of avoiding faecal impaction must be stressed to them. The nurse enquires daily about the bowels, and ensures that when the relatives say there has been an action, they mean an adequate one. If an evacuant suppository is ordered, the nurse stays to see the result.

4. *Keeping the mouth clean and fresh*

A moist tongue and lips contribute a great deal to comfort. While the patient is able to clean his teeth and rinse his mouth he is encouraged to do so. His mouth is inspected regularly; thrush (candidiasis) readily infects the mucous membranes of debilitated people, especially if they have been receiving antibiotics or cytotoxics. Foods such as slivers of pineapple, slices of apple, segments of orange and peeled grapes help to moisten or clean the mouth. Sparkling drinks, such as tonic water, are usually appreciated. Such small delicacies are fairly easily provided in hospital, but can in the home be very expensive— a point discussed later on p. 112.

5. *Giving suitable food and drink*

Although there is no need to press a dying patient to eat, keeping up an adequate fluid intake will improve comfort, keep the mouth moist and prevent acidosis. The use of a feeding cup or drinking straws for those unable to sit up will increase readiness to drink, and for the very weak sips from a teaspoon will moisten the mouth. Many dying people will enjoy very small helpings of food until a very late stage, and relatives like to cook something that is appreciated.

6. *Prevention of pain*

Dying is not invariably associated with pain, and those with pain which cannot be well controlled will usually be transferred to hospital. The nurse must be ready to tell the doctor if pain is not being adequately controlled, so that the analgesic or the dose can be adjusted.

Many hospices print leaflets about the experience they have gained in pain control for the benefit of family doctors. The drugs used, and the principles, are the same as those described for the hospital patient. The dose and the schedule must be calculated so that the patient is free from pain at all times. Regular administration of adequate analgesics is all that is needed; very large doses lead to confusion and deterioration of the personality.

Oral administration is preferable to injections; the effect is slower to manifest itself, but longer lasting and less liable to produce unwanted side-effects. Analgesic suppositories are especially suitable for patients at home. Though the effect may not be so great as by mouth, it is well sustained. A suppository can be inserted last thing at night by the patient or by a relative, and a painfree night may allow both to sleep. Oxycodone pectinate 30 mg is valuable.

Pain is traumatic to the family, who are constantly aware of it, as well as to the patient, and it is essential for the peace of mind of the group that it be effectively controlled.

These aims are shared by the nurse and the family, and their success in achieving them is regularly assessed. The nurse should give approval and praise readily when success is being achieved, and offer advice and clinical help if it is not.

The nurse has other aims; one of the most important is to detect stress in the caring relatives, to discover the causes and to remove or relieve them where possible. When she visits she enquires not only for her patient, but asks the relatives too, 'How are you?' and listens to the answer. Many relatives accept that they are going to have a difficult time and suffer many restrictions in their lives during the final stages of their patient's illness, but find relief in talking about these to a sympathetic listener, and realising that their problems and real sacrifices are understood. People often feel very lonely when their life has narrowed to the care of a single person. Premonitory grief is felt, and also fear about what will happen afterwards. A wife may ask 'What shall I do when he's gone?' She is anticipating the loss of a lifelong companion and also realising that the whole pattern of life is going to change when she no longer has the nursing to do.

Feelings of inadequacy are common; people feel that they ought to be able to deal better with problems of pain or nausea or sleeplessness. Better cooperation from nurse and doctor in identifying difficulties and dealing with them may be indicated. More discussion and reassurance may be needed.

The families of those who are being cared for by the community services of a hospice derive great strength from the knowledge that if their problems are too heavy for them, the patient can be transferred to the hospice. This does not necessarily imply that he will remain there till his death. There may be a specific difficulty about a drug regime to be solved; perhaps all that is needed is a period of rest for the relatives.

It is common to find that one relative, such as a wife or unmarried daughter, is almost entirely responsible for nursing care, and may complain about the burden. It is not unusual to find that, in spite of such complaints, they do not really welcome assistance from others, and that they have a deep need to continue to carry the responsibility. Some, however, are grateful for help in taking a few hours off occasionally to see the shops, get fresh air, and to get out of the house.

Complaints that sleep is disturbed by having to get up at intervals during the night to attend to the sick man are almost universal. Some authorities and services provide for night attendance or night visits which may ameliorate this. The Marie Curie Night Nursing Service provides excellent help for those dying of cancer at home. Sometimes advice can be given about taking an hour or two of sleep after lunch, when the patient can be settled down to sleep as well. If the patient is being wakened by pain, the analgesic may need adjusting. Unpleasant smells are often a problem, more noticeable in the house than in a hospital. They arise mostly from urine and faeces, and from discharges from malignant lesions. Faecal incontinence may result from constipation, and rectal examination should always be made to exclude this as a cause. Incontinence of urine may be relieved by an indwelling catheter, which will give comfort to the patient and the family. Incontinence may be due to confusion, and while this may be caused by cerebral lesions, or mental infirmity, it is sometimes due to an excessive or irregular schedule of analgesics, and may improve when this is corrected. Incontinence pads can be supplied; and many authorities run an incontinence-laundry service which is a boon.

Few lay people realise how offensive the discharge from ulcerating growths can be, and the choice of a dressing to mitigate this may be very helpful. St Barnabas Home, Worthing, recommends the use of live active yoghurt on fungating lesions, for instance, of the breast, as a very effective deodorant. Aserbine may be used if sloughs are present. A drop of 'Dor' or 'Nilodor' on the dressing can neutralise smells. Ordinary household deodorant sprays and tablets for use in bathroom or kitchen are well-known. For use in a sickroom the pine scents are usually more acceptable than 'floral' perfumes.

Caring for a dying person at home invariably means increased expense and sometimes real financial hardship. Many patients feel the cold, so heating bills increase. Food and drinks will include milk, eggs, fruit and cordials, and less of the cheaper filling foods. Additional bed linen may be required. Very often someone has to give up work and stay at home to nurse. If this is a single daughter, it may mean that she is not getting stamps on her insurance cards, and this may have serious effects later on benefit and pension results.

It is important that the family is made aware of all its social entitlements, and makes use of them. A heating allowance and a constant attendance allowance may be available. Commodes, wheelchairs and similar equipment may be obtained on loan from the local authority. Prescription charges can be remitted in suitable cases. The social worker can help the underprivileged to claim social security. Rent rebates are available to many council tenants in difficult circumstances. Voluntary organisations may make gifts, and charitable and religious societies will help their members, such as Jews and Roman Catholics.

There are of course advantages in having a member of the family dying at home rather than in hospital. There is no travel to take up time and money, and the relatives' role is seen clearly as central to the patient's needs, whereas in a hospital they may feel uncertain as to how they can participate. Patients not uncommonly ask to go home, and relatives may feel guilty if they cannot manage this.

It must not be thought that all dying people are easy or

grateful patients. Some are bitter and resentful towards those whom they know are going to be alive after the patient is dead. Sufferers from motor neurone disease, for instance, become aware that they are not having any treatment and that their condition makes inevitable progress. They are still in full command of their intelligence, and may be angry and even show violence to those who care for them. The last scenes may be very traumatic both for patients and relatives. It is quite easy for the nurse to answer anger or abuse with professional courtesy and gentleness, since she suffers no personal pain. She must strive to teach this attitude to the family, if it is required.

After the death of someone in a ward, it is not usual for the nurse to see the family again, and so their needs then and later are unknown to her. In the community this is much less likely; the home nurse is likely to meet the family, or to attend some other member. The experience that they have shared is a bond between them and post-bereavement visits should be paid by the community nurses.

The Funeral

The doctor provides the death certificate, and also a notice for the relatives giving some information on the formalities that have to be undertaken. This certificate has to be presented to the registrar of births and deaths who will issue the certificate which allows the funeral to take place. The registrar will also usually give advice about the need for copies of the death certificate, e.g. for friendly societies or banks, and what to do about pension books.

The first thing that relatives have to do is to choose an undertaker or funeral director, and the doctor or nurse may be asked to make a suggestion, though when death is expected the family will probably have thought about this. The undertaker has a very important role in making the occasion as painless as possible, and many of them are very conscious of their social function, and of the comfort and support they can give.

When someone has died at home, he may remain there until the funeral. The undertaker finds out the wishes of the family about a coffin, brings it, prepares the body and later fastens up the coffin. It is increasingly common, however, for the body to be removed at once to a funeral home, especially in crowded urban conditions.

There are many decisions to be made, the first one being whether there is to be burial or cremation. For cremation, an additional certificate by a second doctor is required. Once the undertaker has the certificate, the date and time of the funeral can be arranged with the vicar and the cemetery or crematorium. The undertaker enquires about the need to send notices to the national or local press, whether flowers are to be accepted, and whether a wedding ring or other jewellery is to be left on the body. The priest or minister will call to offer condolences and arrange the type of service.

A funeral is a great expense, and among the old there is a lot of anxiety about how bills are to be met. A death grant is payable to an insured person and his dependents; this has stood at £30 since 1969, and bears no relation to actual costs, which in 1980 were not below £400. Even this £30 is not payable to the very old, who have not made the requisite insurance contribution.

While lavish displays are now thought by many to be unsuitable, the value to the mourners of a suitable expression of their feelings at parting must not be underestimated. It may be worth recalling the way funerals were always conducted for ordinary people until quite recently. Flowers and wreaths arrived at the house, blinds were drawn in neighbours' houses, the hearse arrived with cars for the mourners, the coffin was borne out with the flowers and the cortege went to the church, with men raising their hats as they passed. The coffin was taken into the church, and the service for the burial of the dead, with its memorable words, took place. Coffin, priest and mourners then went to the cemetery for the interment. It was an occasion from which mourners could draw memories of words and images to comfort them.

In cities it is now more common for mourners to meet at the crematorium chapel. One commitment has just ended, another will begin as soon as this one is finished. Those who have a circle of friends and colleagues may be remembered later in the service of thanksgiving, which has replaced the memorial service. For most bereaved families the service in the chapel is all they have to remember.

There are, of course, optional expenses which may be incurred. In Ireland it is still common in the country to hold a 'Wake' before burial, when mourners gather to drink to the memory of the deceased and to talk about him. Mourning clothes are not very generally worn nowadays. Headstones and memorials of various kinds are also less common than formerly. The decision not to use them may have to be taken quite early, since many local authorities lay out their cemeteries as 'lawns', and stonework is not permitted.

The rituals attendant on death are of great importance in determining how bereaved people feel afterwards, and to provide them with something on which to fix their thoughts, and to store in their hearts in pictures and words. Nurses who are asked to go to the funeral of their patients are receiving a great honour.

Some elderly people have no relatives, and the local authority will pay the funeral expenses, and recover these from the patient's estate.

It will be seen that the time from the death to the funeral involves a lot of emotional events, culminating in the final act of consignment to earth or to fire. Following this comes a time of emotional anticlimax and painful duties and perhaps decisions. Since women usually live longer than men, one often finds it is a widow who has to dispose of her husband's clothes and perhaps the tools of his trade. She has to decide where she is going to live, and will be well advised not to make decisions under the immediate stress of her loss.

She also has to think about her way of life and her attitude to widowhood; and she may feel in her first grief that, having cooked and cared for her husband, and perhaps tired from his last illness, that she has lost the incentive to make efforts on her own behalf. This is the time when the counsel and support of the community nurse can be valuable. If a woman has children or friends around her, it is easy to find a reason for containing grief and thinking of others. For isolates it is less easy, but she should be urged to keep up morale, take a good diet, take care of grooming, and look for opportunities to give to others. All of us have some function in the later stages of our lives; we may have the resources and abilities to do things for others. All of us fear dependence and loss of faculties, but we must not allow grief to bring about this state unnecessarily. It is the lot of some people who decline into helplessness to give others the opportunity to display compassion and caring. Bereavement should not bring this state nearer by self-neglect or indifference.

Sudden Death at Home

An unexpected death of someone who was not known to be ill, and who has not been seen by his own doctor within the last month may occur at home. The doctor should be summoned to confirm that death has occurred, but he will be unable to supply the death certificate because he cannot state the cause of death. He rings the local coroner, and an official from the coroner's court will soon arrive.

The representative will explain (e.g. to a wife after a husband's death) what is going to happen. He looks at the patient for any unusual circumstances, removes any jewellery or watches and gives them to the wife for safe-keeping. He explains that the patient must be examined to find the cause of death, avoiding unpleasant terms like 'post-mortem' or 'autopsy'. This examination may take a little time, especially in a busy urban practice, and he indicates the earliest date for which funeral arrangements will be feasible. He has a good local knowledge of local funeral directors, and can suggest a few firms. If the family attends a church or chapel, they will know the name of the minister they want to officiate, but again suitable names can be offered by the coroners clerk.

He then contacts the undertaker selected, and asks them to effect a coroner's removal; that is, that they will take the deceased to the coroner's court for autopsy. This removal can be rather traumatic in a small flat or house, and the relatives are advised to retire to a neighbour's, or to a closed room until it has been completed.

Once the cause of death has been found to be a natural one, the burial certificate can be issued and the funeral arrangements made.

11

The dying child and the family

The most dangerous time for a baby is before he is born, and immediately afterwards; the mortality rate drops sharply after the first fortnight. In Western countries we are so much better able to preserve life that the death of a child causes special concern. There are, however, many parts of the world where such death is so common that it is an event that afflicts all families, and is attended by resignation rather than with strong emotion.

The causes of infant mortality change markedly over the years. Death from infectious disease, such a terrible scourge in the last century, is becoming noticeably less common, and this means that other causes become proportionately more important. Cancer has now become as common as infection in causing death in the 5- to 10-year-old age group and accidents now rank as the most frequent cause. This term covers injuries received at home or on the roads and preventive medicine has a role of very great possibility in reducing this sad figure.

The principles of nursing care for child victims of serious injury are those followed in all trauma cases and will not be further considered here. The parents, however, when they lose a child through injury have not only endured a quite unexpected loss, but are customarily racked with guilt and remorse. The best parents often suffer the most; mothers continually reproach themselves for having turned their back on a child for a moment or two. Fathers who were driving the car involved in an accident, even if blameless, feel that they should not have taken that road, or at that time, even though they realise that nothing could be done to avert the accident.

There are of course instances in which one or both parents are to blame, and nurses caring for an injured child in such circumstances may well feel this. They are, however, not in the position of being able to judge what is right and, even if they were, should not express reproach but offer such support as they can. Guilt, real or imaginary, and its consequences will be discussed again a little later in connection with deaths from other causes.

Malignant disease accounts for about a fifth of all deaths of children between 5- and 10-years-old. Some of these conditions now respond to treatment and quite long periods of remission, if not cure, can now be obtained by surgery, radiotherapy and chemotherapy. In others no such treatment is effective.

Children Dying of Malignant Disease

The principles of physical care for children with cancer is closely related to that of adults, as far as relief of symptoms goes.

Pain is felt and must be prevented if possible rather than merely relieved. Children express rapidly and vehemently their reaction to pain, and this is distressing not only for the patient, but also his ward-mates, relatives and nurses. Drugs by mouth are much preferable to injections, which most children detest and fear. Stopping active treatment when there is no hope of cure may be a relief for parents and patient because it means an end to injections.

The mixture of oral drugs used for adults must be greatly modified for children. It is best not to use cocaine, which makes children tense and prone to muscle twitching. Paediatric staff accustomed to treating malignant disease believe that morphine is greatly superior to diamorphine in a pain-relieving mixture. It must not be started before other less powerful drugs have been used, and the principles of regular dosage, and not allowing pain to become established hold good in these instances.

Like adults, children may become constipated if they are

enfeebled, and morphine is being given, but although it must be watched for, it is very much less common than in adults. Retention of urine and faeces does not enter into a child's view of physiology. Pressure sores too may occur, and the usual precautions about position, and preventing and relieving pressure must be followed.

Appetite is variable, but often good, especially if the mother can help with the cooking of snacks, and there is no need to put any restrictions on the child's fancies. If the mother is to be allowed to go into the kitchen to fry a sausage, the kitchen staff as well as the nurses must be tolerant and accepting, and kindly, concerned domestic staff are vital to the good conduct of a paediatric ward. To help like this affords the mother a role, and prevents feelings of helplessness. She can give drinks and measure them, and the ability to give food to her child is a very basic need.

Occupation and company should be provided for a child up to the end, or unnecessary boredom results. Children should never be compelled to undertake activity, but there is rarely any need to prevent them. In one paediatric ward a regular week-day employment of the children who were up and about was to make biscuits, jam tarts and aptly-named rock cakes for tea. This was greatly enjoyed, and even children not far from death would want to join in. If children are being nursed at home they will join in many activities, and there is no need to restrict them because they are in hospital. If they wish to be taken to the zoo, or for a ride, requests should be seriously considered and can be granted. The general attitude should be 'Why not?' rather than a refusal.

Justin contracted a sarcoma of the upper end of the humerus when he was 10. He had radiotherapy, but there was recurrence at the site, and when he was 14 a forequarter amputation was performed. The operation did not halt the disease and it was evident that Justin's illness was terminal. He was a serious, intelligent boy, deeply interested in planes, and with a special attachment to Concorde. Some of the Hospital Friends arranged a trip for him to Heathrow, where he was taken aboard Concorde, and sat in the right-hand seat in the cockpit while the pilot gave him a technical description of take-off procedure. He talked incessantly about this and listened on a radio to pilot-talk until he died.

Pedro was approaching his fifth birthday and was not going to have another one. His parents told Sister that they had bought him a white miniature poodle for his birthday which would be waiting for him when he got home. Sister said 'Why not bring it up and show Pedro on his birthday?'. The dog came up in a basket, and it gave the little boy immense pleasure. This visit was repeated each Saturday afternoon until Pedro died.

'Occupation' need not mean doing anything very active; it may be reading or looking at pictures, or drawing or merely lying and listening to mother. When parents are absent, some undemanding company from a nurse is much appreciated. Attending the hospital school should be allowed if the child wants to be present, though demands on him are not made other than to attend, not to do any real work.

Older children and teenagers have less expectation than infants about the continuous presence of parents; they may express understanding that parents have other commitments, and even feel they need a little time of their own to join in ward activities. Although this is an age when relations with parents are difficult, through struggles to uphold their own rights, these disputes rarely appear in serious or terminal illness. As teenagers become more ill they become more dependent, and welcome their parents' presence.

What should children be told?

Children encounter death in various ways and usually at quite an early age. Pets die, and the child's grief is often much lessened by a funeral in the garden. Grandparents may die, and their death and burial may be equated with those of pets. Children have in general a simple, straightforward view of death that includes a belief in a very substantial after-life. If parents are agnostics it is sometimes hard to know where these beliefs come from, but schoolfellows and friends and picture books are usual sources. Few parents could bring themselves to say to a child whose tortoise has just been buried that it has gone forever. The usual story is that it has gone to heaven, and the child speedily gets a feeling for a heaven that is peopled with canaries, goldfish and grandmothers. They do not in general think of joining them, but have a matter of fact attitude.

Robin's five-year-old friend had died in an accident. He questioned his mother as to where he was, and she answered 'He's gone to be with Jesus'. 'Oh' said Robin with relief 'I know Him' and asked no more.

Most people agree in theory if not in practice that adults should know that they are going to die, if they ask. Most professionals would hesitate to say the same about children. In a ward where children with malignant disease are being treated, it is inevitable that children will die, and children are so mobile in most paediatric wards that they all know each other. If a child dies in the night, when the lights go up, the smaller children ask the night nurse, 'Where's John?' She usually answers 'He's gone; yes, he's gone away; yes, his Mummy was with him'. Children are used to others going to other wards, or theatres and make no further comment. Older ones and teenagers do not ask, and if they are seen at all as a group, it may be wise to say 'I expect you know John has died, but I though it better not to say so to the little ones'. The teenagers usually say 'Yes, they did know'.

Nurses are sometimes asked by a child if he is going to die, or perhaps more often, is he ever going to get better? This is usually from a younger child — older ones do not often ask. Perhaps they have a good idea about what is happening, but prefer not to have it brought into the open. The same phenomenon has been noticed in adults who find it easier to behave normally without having to discuss their approaching end.

Sometimes there is a slightly indirect approach; an older child may ask in connection with one who has died, 'Have I got the same thing wrong with me?' The answer to this is normally a truthful 'No'. There are so many different kinds of growth, or of lymphadenopathy, of mode of onset and of extent of spread, that it would be wrong to say that a child's condition was exactly the same as another's. Junior nurses should be encouraged to talk with sister about this way of approaching questions.

Having said all this, there will be times when a nurse is asked a direct question. This is a story recalled by an experienced paediatric sister about the first time she was asked this question, by a seven year old.

'Am I going to die, Sister?'

'I don't know; nobody knows, but I don't think we can make you well'.

'Does my mother know?'

'She doesn't know any more than I do'.

'Shall I see my grandmother in heaven'.

'Yes, surely'.

'What about Pussy?'

'Yes, I think so'.

Short pause — then,

'Is it nearly supper time?'

Family Support for the Bereaved

Mothers, fathers and grandparents all react in their own individual way to loss of a child, and express (or do not express) their grief in various ways. Guilt has been alluded to in cases of accident, but occurs also in connection with cancer. Most people know nowadays that X-rays and smoking are associated in different ways with malignant disease. Parents may ask, could it be that my chest X-ray had anything to do with it? Fathers may accuse the mother of smoking during pregnancy. Mothers may allude to the father smoking in the living room or polluting the atmosphere. Professionals must try hard and at once to eradicate guilt, which if it is entertained for long will become an entrenched belief and may lead to a break-up of the marriage. It is sad that the loss of a child sometimes seems to act as a catalyst in a variety of ways to the separation of the parents.

Parents may also project this feeling of guilt on to others, blaming doctors and nurses for what they feel is slow diagnosis or ineffective treatment. Nurses should of course take all complaints seriously, but must not allow themselves to be disturbed by criticism they feel to be unjustified. Nurses may answer that they understand parents' feelings, but they think they will come to understand that everyone has done the best they can.

Many observers think that three years is about the time it takes to come to terms with a loss, and that it differs between the two partners, or if there are other children, and both parents of different ages. Some long for support and welcome social workers and health visitors who care to call. It is easy to allow the bereaved to become over-dependent and it must be recognised that there is an ideal or compromise time when support is progressively withdrawn.

There are many different modes of reaction, but a not uncommon one is for parents to throw themselves into schemes for raising money for cancer research and similar projects. While the general principle is admirable, some schemes are not entirely wise. Parents may want to raise funds for a scanner or such apparatus for the hospital in which their child died when there is already similar apparatus at a neighbouring hospital.

The bereaved mother's problems are in one way more severe than the husband's. If the dead child was an only one, she will be left at home alone while he goes out to work. She is too dispirited to join much with neighbours, who in some circles are reluctant to let their children go to the house where a child had a malignant disease for fear of 'catching something'.

If there are no other pre-school children, the mother may be encouraged to take a part-time job or voluntary work which will mean that she is not alone all day in the house.

When a child dies, the parents may strip his room and dispose of his belongings at once. They hope to shorten the period of mourning, but life does not yet work like this. On the other hand, some parents keep this room and his belongings intact for long periods, claiming that they feel unable to do anything or that throwing out things is tantamount to throwing out his memory.

Sooner or later these parents may ask, 'Is it time to clear the room?' Nurses need express no other opinion than a guarded optimism; the question indicates that the parents are approaching the solution to the problem.

As most people do, we have primarily been considering the

plight of the bereaved mother, but that of the father is often disregarded.

> Mr and Mrs Y. were middle-class professional people who had lost their younger child, a girl with a very disfiguring malignant disease. She had not any symptoms that could not be controlled, but her parents had a very harrowing time. They were a close, affectionate couple.
>
> One day Mr Y. came in from work, put his elbows on the tea-table and began to cry. His wife feared some disaster at work, but eventually he said that everyone asked him how she was, and no one seemed to think that he too had feelings and problems, and was desolate with grief. They were a loving pair who, when she was more aware of his problems, could help with them.

If there are other children, their needs must be thought about constantly. Unless one child was exceedingly close to the dead one, the children's problems tend to be those of the parents, rather than inherent in the children. Parents must not allow their own problems to burden the children. Neither is it wise to refuse to mention death or the missing unit to children —they may fear that there is some mystery or discreditable fact about it that they do not understand.

> Pat was seven when her aunt died. This was Muriel, a beautiful, gay, sweet-scented figure of life to Pat, who learned later that her aunt had tuberculosis. Aunt Muriel was never alluded to, never spoken about, because it was felt that Pat was too young to know about death.
>
> Pat was very fond of her aunt and could not understand this silence. She felt that there must be something disgraceful about the sudden disappearance of her aunt. She learned the facts later, but never forgot the pain and confusion the episode cost her.

Bereaved Children

It is relatively more common for children to lose a parent than for parents to lose a child, and has different problems. First there are those of coming to terms with death and coming to some solution acceptable to them with regard to death and life after death.

Children do not think in the same way as adults do and will accept simplistic and magic solutions that they may smile over when adults.

> Mrs N. was a middle-aged lady who lost her husband suddenly. Her daughter had two little girls, aged 5 and 7, who spent a night with their grandmother when the parents wanted to go out to dinner. The children woke early, and came to grandmother and got into bed with her with much pleasure. The younger said, 'We mustn't leave grandfather out in the cold', and got up and took his photograph from the dressing table and got into bed again with it.

The other factor, with which bereaved children have to come to terms with, is the fact that the remaining parent may acquire a new partner, and the children a step-parent. Women can usually cope better alone than men, in that running a house comes more easily than to most men, but find it more difficult to get well-paid employment. However, it must be emphasised that the new member of the household is usually well-accepted by the child and normally does well as a surrogate parent.

12

Problems and predicaments

In writing the preceding chapters on the care of the family in which a death is going to occur, much time and thought has been spent on practical details. The choice of drugs, the relief of symptoms, the reactions to be expected, the statutory aspects. These are what nurses want to know, when they ask — 'How can I help?' 'What can I say?' 'What must I do?'

In supplying such information, one must not be dogmatic. One does not always say or do the right thing; the most devoted and caring team may sometimes feel when they evaluate their care after the death of a patient that their aims for him and his family did not turn out as well as had been hoped. We must not ignore such events, neither must we be unduly cast down. We must aim by thought and consultation with colleagues and by listening to others to qualify ourselves in every way for the work we are doing. We may sometimes say, 'We did as best we knew'; but add, 'Is it possible to increase our knowledge and skill?'

Not everyone will agree with the views expressed on some topics, for instance, the belief that truthfulness in dealing with the dying is of fundamental importance. By no means all doctors would conform to this in practice, and for a variety of reasons. They may feel that the time is not ripe, and honestly believe that a soothing or cheery lie is in the patient's best interests. Some doctors would deny that a verdict of approaching death should ever be given to a patient and that their function is to sustain hope to the end. Instead, most of these doctors would tell the relatives.

Neither must it be presumed that an answer that is truthful is appropriate, or even a correct answer to what the patient is saying. If a man with an early carcinoma of colon asks 'Have I got cancer?' it would be true to answer 'Yes', but it would be better in every sense to say 'You have a growth that we can treat, and probably treat successfully'. What the patient means by his question is, 'Am I going to die soon?' and the answer is almost certainly 'No'.

Junior nurses do not have the knowledge to give a good answer in most cases to questions about the prognosis of cancers. New treatments are introduced, the outlook in many conditions is improved, and there may be many factors about the extent of the growth and the patient's general condition that will influence the answer.

Once a diagnosis of a malignant condition has been made, it may be wrong to allow the patient to believe he will die soon; in many cases treatment will produce remission, and years of useful life, or even cure.

> Mr T. was a solicitor in a Midland town, with a wife and two children aged 6 and 8 years. He came to the oncological ward of a London hospital after a short illness, and was diagnosed as suffering from acute leukaemia. He had read some accounts of this, and was anxious and depressed about his future. He asked the registrar, 'Am I wrong to hope?'. The answer to this is of course, 'No'. There are methods today of treating leukaemia which are effective for quite long periods, and the survival rate improves constantly. Apart from this, the longer a man lives, the greater is the possibility of a big advance in knowledge and a breakthrough in treatment. One can instance diabetes mellitus, once a fatal disease. Mr T. may indeed hope.
>
> It was in fact four years later that Mr T. reached a stage when it was judged time to discontinue efforts at cure, and to treat only his symptoms. He had had four years of happy family life, had made prudent arrangements about his affairs, and the children were that much older. He did not at this stage ask if he should hope, because he knew. Had he asked, it would be judged by most people to be wrong, when he was a week or so from death, to suggest that he might recover.

Persistence in denying to a dying patient that there is no hope of recovery is sometimes defended as being 'kind' to him. Doctors and nurses may genuinely believe that this is their motive, but must be aware that sometimes they have a desire to avoid the complications of admitting that death is inevitable. It may mean difficult conversations with patient and family. There may be emotions raised, questions asked, requests made for further opinions. These are disturbing to the medical staff, who can avoid them by refusing to admit that death is approaching. Our function is to cure and give life, and it is disturbing to have to admit failure. We must try to ensure that our reasons either for giving or withholding information are good ones.

Mr R. had been admitted to a surgical ward with acute intestinal obstruction. He was well-known to the surgeon and the ward sister, having had two operations in the preceding year. The first was for excision of a growth of the transverse colon; the second was because of adhesions to the resection site. Laparotomy on this occasion revealed extensive secondary peritoneal deposits and inoperable carcinomatosis. He was returned to the ward to a sideroom, with an intravenous infusion and an intranasal gastric tube. The surgeon came in that evening, and visited Mr R. with the ward sister, a colleague of long standing. The patient was awake and painfree, and asked the surgeon quietly, 'Am I going to die?' The surgeon was not expecting the question, and after a perceptible pause, answered with a smile, 'No, no, everything will be all right'. Outside in the corridor he stopped and said to the Sister, 'I ought to have told him the truth'. He thought for a little and then said, 'I would go back and tell him, but it would make me look so silly'. The Sister said, 'I agree with you that this is the time', and he went back and spent some time alone with the patient. Mr R. told the Sister when she went back what relief and peace he felt, and that he was looking forward to a full, frank talk with his wife.

Problems of Medication

The principles of relieving pain by drugs in terminal illness have been worked out mainly in hospices, and in theory this knowledge is available to all medical staff. Pain is prevented, rather than relieved, by regular adequate dosage, first by simple analgesics, then by the more powerful ones. The opiates are started when they are needed, but not earlier, so that very large doses are not required. If drugs are used with less skill through lack of experience, it is possible to have a patient receiving very large doses of morphine, but still anxious, demanding, and complaining of pain. This is disturbing to staff and to relatives as well. The remedy might be wider dissemination of knowledge already possessed by hospices. Nurses who are called upon to give doses in excess of the theoretical maximum are often disturbed usually because they feel they are being asked to shorten the patient's life. This occurs in circumstances where the management of the drug regime has been injudicious, and communication between doctors and nurses is not a two-way one. Both groups should feel able to explain to the other what their aims are, and how they are thinking and feeling.

The following is a quotation from *Moral Dilemmas in Medicine* by a nurse who had been asked by a surgeon to give 50 mg of diamorphine to a patient with terminal cancer.

> 'To end the patient's life was against all my upbringing, my nursing conscience and my religious convictions. But . . . if I refused to give the injection that might be the end of my career in general nursing.' (Campbell, A.V. *Moral Dilemmas in Medicine*. (Churchill Livingstone)

There is something wrong with most aspects of this sad situation. The use of analgesics for this unfortunate patient had evidently been badly managed. The surgeon was quite wrong to ask a nurse to give a dose of this order, and especially because he apparently ordered this verbally and not in writing. It is sad that the nurse felt unable to voice her feeling at once to the surgeon, and sadder still that she felt (even without justification) that she would be victimised, and that this weighed against her moral convictions.

What eventually happened in this case we do not know. The basic lack of communication and understanding between doctor and nurse cannot be easily remedied. If the nurse had consulted a nursing officer, it is to be hoped that she reminded the surgeon that drug orders must be in writing, and asked if he would write the dose on the drug sheet and sign his name. If he declines to do so, the nurse cannot proceed with the injection.

Patients who are receiving regular analgesics for terminal

pain will be getting quite large doses, and eventually will die of their disease, but not of the drugs used to control pain. Nevertheless, nurses sometimes fear being the one who gives the injection before death, as if they were responsible for death. The programme of drugs should be discussed by sister with all her nurses, noticing how effective it is, and placing the emphasis on pain control and not on the approach of death. Seniors should not repeat to juniors this old feeling about giving the last injection. All the team are responsible for devising and carrying out a good plan for the patient's comfort, and have a joint responsibility. It is easy to understand and sympathise with this attitude about the administration of large doses of analgesic. There are many tales and superstitions which are still told in the country. Owls hoot outside windows, the death watch beetle is heard, a bird flies down the chimney, coffin handles form on wax candles, clocks stop unexpectedly. These are not likely to occur in hospital, but some nurses still believe that having lilies in the ward or combining red with white flowers will cause a death in the ward within forty-eight hours. In all occupations and professions stories are passed on from seniors to new recruits, but it is time that this one faded out.

In connection with the evaluation of the results of care described in the use of the nursing process, it is important to discuss after the death of the patient how successful the plan had been in ensuring a calm and peaceful end, from the standpoint of patient, relatives and staff. Sister should encourage contributions from junior nurses. The nursing report exchange is the usual time for such discussions, but a ward meeting in which the doctor is involved should not neglect to review the success or otherwise of management.

The Extent of Responsibility

The amount of responsibility for continuing care of bereaved families is not universally accepted. Doctors have tended in recent years to accept functions of caring for the depressed, the anxious, the guilty, and the socially inferior, that would once have been thought the province of the priest. Some feel that they do not have the time or training to shoulder the emotional problems of all their patients and their families.

The concept of care implicit in hospice medicine will probably tend to increase the willingness to undertake some responsibility for the bereaved. Nurses in hospital rarely see any relatives again, but community nurses and health visitors know these problems well. They not only listen to stories of grief but can give practical advice to those deprived of the help of a life-partner. Many general practitioners play a very important role in giving comfort.

> A country practitioner had been in hospital and off work for a fortnight following a fracture. During this time two of the elderly patients in his practice had died and on his return to work he visited both homes. One widow spoke with gratitude of his call, his expression of liking for his former patient, and his sympathy. 'He's a real doctor', she commented.

Euthanasia

Bona mors, the good death, has been the desire of man and the aim of his nurses for centuries, and this book has endeavoured to described how through professional skill and knowledge we can help to bring this about. Euthanasia means literally no more than 'a good death', but it is now applied by common usage to the termination of life, either by the hand of the patient himself or of another, when it is judged (again either by the patient or by others) that life is intolerable and that death is preferable.

The arguments in favour of and against euthanasia have been conducted for years in literature, in the press, and in the legislative. In a book which aims to describe practical care, it does not seem appropriate to examine exhaustively the issues and arguments put forward. It is however necessary to point out the legal aspects involved, and to draw attention to the authors' beliefs. Both are Christians, members of the Church of England, and do not accept the arguments of those who favour euthanasia. It is however also necessary to point out that there are on both sides people who take an extreme position, and also people of compassion and concern. In the bibliography are references to organisations devoted to the propagation of belief in euthanasia. It must not be thought that either side has the monopoly of sympathy and feeling for the distress of others.

Suicide

Suicide is as old as recorded history, and is the subject of
rather unreal and idealistic views by those who have no
practical association with its problems and consequences, as
nurses and doctors do. Socrates drinking the hemlock is
thought of as dying with calm and dignity, and the symptoms
of his last act are not considered. Keats thought of it as 'to
cease upon the midnight with no pain', but there is no way of
assuring such an end by suicide. Senior nurses will recall the
days when drinking corrosive poisons was not an uncommon
method. Coal–gas poisoning was comparatively simple for
the suicide, but involved danger to innocent neighbours.
Those of us who live in London and travel regularly on the
Underground Railway must have heard the chilling
announcement of delay 'due to a person under a train'.

Suicide used to be a criminal offence, but has not been so
since 1961. Those of us who work in Casualty Department, or
read the newspapers, cannot fail to gather painful impres-
sions about suicide. They learn of young people making inef-
fectual efforts, perhaps intentionally so; of gifted people des-
troying themselves when in acute depression; of dreadful
violence inflicted on the person; of people who believe, often
groundlessly, that they have cancer. We often hear people say
that life is not worth living or that they wish they were dead,
but these appear to be the middle-aged or elderly equivalent
of the swallowing of a few aspirin tablets by a teenager. They
are pleas for help, that life should be less painful or less
lonely. It is not really a plea that life should be ended for them.

If those suffering from pain or incapacitating disease wish
to end their lives, there are organisations that sympathise
with this wish as expressed. The Voluntary Euthanasia Society, now renamed Exit, is the chief one in the United King-
dom. This Society recognises that if suicide is to be effective,
would-be clients must receive some information and instruction about methods. The Scottish Euthanasia Society published in 1980 a booklet, 'How to Die with Dignity', available
in theory to those who had been members of the Society for
two years. In fact, it very soon was made available to the press
and freely quoted (e.g. *The Listener*, 18th September, 1980, p.
363). It is obvious that this material can soon be read by

depressives and by young people, and that there is no way in which this knowledge, once in print, can be kept confined to those for whom it is intended. It is an offence to assist someone to commit suicide, however altruistic one's motives may be. Many people will feel that this provision is a protection to many old people, who feel they are a burden to families or nurses, or can be made to feel so.

The dangers and problems of this subject were well illustrated in the press reports and the prosecution and conviction of two members of the staff of Exit in 1981 for assisting would-be suicides. It was evident that some of the requests for euthanasia were from temporarily depressed people who were frightened when they were confronted with the possibility of death.

The suggestions about suicide are meant to be an acceptable alternative to a restricted life. Their advocates point to geriatric hospitals, and say the existence offered there is intolerable. If so, this is a reason for improving the standard of care, and we invite critics to come and help us rather than merely offer means of suicide. Many patients in such hospitals are not capable of forming a real intention and for these a rather more sinister programme is advocated. If they are unable to commit suicide, they should be helped to do so, presumably by doctors and nurses.

Clinical Euthanasia

The legalisation of euthanasia, requested by a patient and carried out by doctors and nurses, or other appointed people, has been from time to time proposed, and bills introduced into Parliament. The last attempt was in 1976, when the proposal was debated and decisively defeated in the House of Lords. The Criminal Law Revision Committee has also considered creating a special kind of homicide, the popularly named 'mercy killing', but turned it down.

There are two points against such laws. The first is that most doctors and nurses are deeply reluctant to undertake to make a decision as to whether a request for death is truly voluntary, and even more reluctant to execute such a decision.

The other factor is that many of the people whom Exit

would regard as leading into. ble lives are incapable of making any decision about it, an t is only a small step from voluntary euthanasia to sanitary measures designed to dispose of these people. Once this has been conceded, it might be thought that not only the old, but the young who were grossly handicapped, either mentally or physically, might also be assisted out of this world. Such views have been publicly expressed in print and in Parliament.

There is, of course, no way of knowing how time and circumstances may modify professional views. At the beginning of the century the therapeutic abortion rate of the 1980s would have been totally unacceptable and it has been widely held that acceptance of abortion would eventually result in acceptance of euthanasia for the elderly in poor physical condition. This has not yet happened, but one cannot be sure. In the event of an atomic explosion in a city, there would be many casualties for whom treatment was hopeless, and to whom none could be offered. Might we feel that these could be offered euthanasia? Few people would like to give a quick answer.

It behoves us all to think, as well as to feel, about our profession and the responsibilities that it entails. If life seems intolerable to some of our patients, the answer may be to seek to improve the quality of that life, rather than to end it.

Experienced sisters have all at some time or other heard appeals from relatives who say something like 'How much longer is it going to last? I don't feel I can stand much more'. It may be that relatives have a right to be considered, but if their ability to cope, and not that of the patient, is the criterion the idea of euthanasia as being voluntary no longer applies. The answer is to try to find out what it is that the relatives cannot bear, and to try to relieve it. Perhaps pain control is not adequate. If the patient is being nursed at home, relatives may have severe problems about sleep, or money, and perhaps it is time to transfer the patient elsewhere, or to get more assistance.

One tendency that must be resisted is to speak of old and helpless people in general terms instead of as individuals. They are spoken of by some as geriatrics, a demeaning term; nobody speaks of a child as a paediatric. Sometimes they are alluded to as vegetables or cabbages, a cruel and degrading practice, with no element of truth in it, except that they cannot speak to defend themselves. Once we think of old people as cabbages, we shall feel that they need nothing except to be watered and set out in rows.

The following story is of a very old lady who died after several years in a long-stay geriatric ward.

Mrs L. was a 95-year-old lady who had been admitted to a continuing care geriatric ward five years before. She had fallen at home and fractured her femur. Although this had healed well, it had caused an upset in her general condition. She had been mildly confused at home, but after her fall she became and remained very confused. She would answer simple questions about herself in a high pitched whisper, but she did not know where she was, what time of day it was or what year it was. She also had diabetes mellitus which was controlled by a 150 g carbohydrate diet and oral chlorpropamide 250 mg daily. Although she never had more than a trace of sugar in her urine, her blood sugar level, which was checked regularly by the doctor, remained moderately high indicating the need to continue her diet and oral medication.

Mrs L. was a thin lady, but she loved her meals. Due to cerebellar degeneration over the last two years, she had little control over her limbs and therefore she needed feeding by the nurses. She was unable to walk and spent each day either up and dressed in a chair, or in bed on a ripple mattress as she was 'at risk' on the Norton Scale (Table 1, p. 34). She was incontinent of urine and therefore had a permanent catheter. This was changed regularly once a month on the date indicated on her care plan. The nurses also aimed to get her to drink 1500 ml of fluid a day to prevent a urinary tract infection. She made no spontaneous conversation and her only enjoyment seemed to be at mealtimes, and when she was given diabetic chocolate, which she loved, in between meals.

Mrs L's only son occasionally visited, and during one of these visits he told the nurse looking after her that Mrs L. enjoyed singing gospel songs when she was younger. This was noted on her care plan, and the nurses would place her near the radio or television when gospel songs were played. She always responded by becoming wreathed in smiles, but she never said anything or tried to join in with the singing.

Two months after her 95th birthday Mrs L. seemed unwell to the nurses. Her uncontrolled limb movements were quieter and her appetite was less. Although she ate her breakfast it was

with less enthusiasm than usual. She had no rise of temperature and there were no other signs of infection. She was washed
and dressed after breakfast and sat out in her chair. However,
an hour later she was slumped in a corner of her chair and it was
decided to put her back to bed. She refused her lunch— a most
unusual occurrence. The doctor examined her but could find no
definite cause for her deterioration except 'old age'. The ward
sister contacted her son to tell him of Mrs L's weak condition.
Mrs L. continued to go downhill, refusing all nourishment and
sleeping most of the time. Although the nurses felt sad about
Mrs L's deterioration as some of them had cared for her for
several years they understood that she was now dying in a
natural way. Mrs L. rallied a little when her son arrived and
smiled in recognition as he approached her bedside. He stayed
with her for an hour or so, and soon after he left Mrs L. lapsed
into unconsciousness. She was turned from side-to-side every
two hours and her mouth was kept moist and clean. She died
peacefully in the early hours of the following morning. The
night sister rang her son just before she went off duty at 7.30
a.m.

It would be possible, by selecting some aspects of Mrs L's
physical and mental condition during her last years, to give an
account which would lead those who believe in euthanasia to
cite her as an example of someone leading an intolerable life,
who ought to be relieved of it.

Quite a different story could, however, be extracted. This
old lady until the last day of her life enjoyed her food, liked
chocolate and listening to the radio, and recognised her son
with pleasure. The nurses 'felt sad' as her end approached;
they did not feel relief at no longer having to undertake her
total care. Her son had the satisfaction of having been faithful
until her death.

If we feel that some old patient nearing the end of life is
withdrawn from our understanding and reach, we should
look at the history, and remember that this was a craftsman,
or the mother of a family, with years of work for society to
their credit. Let us recall that we are now being offered
through the bodies of the old and the dying an opportunity to
increase the amount of compassion and loving kindness in
the world. We must remember our aims in nursing every
dying patient, to achieve a painfree and fitting end and that
until that time they should be enabled to pass their days in
rest and quietness.

Bibliography

General

Browning, M.H., Lewis, E.P. (1972). *The Dying Patient: A Nursing Perspective*. New York: The American Journal of Nursing.
Hinton, J. (1967). *Dying*. Harmondsworth: Penguin Books.
Kübler-Ross, E. (1969). *On Death and Dying*. London: Tavistock Publications.
Lamerton, R. (1980). *Care of the Dying*. Harmondsworth: Penguin Books.
Nursing Mirror (1974). Symposium — Care of the dying. *Nursing Mirror*, **139**, Oct 10; pp. 53–70.
Nursing Times (1980). *Care of the Terminal Patient*. London: Macmillan Journals.
Raven, R.W., ed. (1975). *The Dying Patient*. Tunbridge: Pitman Medical.
Saunders, C. (1976). *Care of the Dying* (Nursing Times Publication). London: Macmillan Journals.
Saunders, C., ed. (1978). *The Management of Terminal Disease*. London: Edward Arnold.

Religious

Autton, N. (1978). *Peace at the Last*. London: S.P.C.K. (Christian view.)
Baqui, M.A. (1979). Muslim teaching concerning death. *Nursing Times* (Occasional Paper) **75**, 10; pp. 43/44.
Formby, J. (1978). Christian teaching concerning death; a Roman Catholic approach. *Nursing Times* (Occasional Paper); **74**, 15; pp. 58–59.
Gordon Jones, A. (1978). Christian teaching concerning death — a non-conformist approach. *Nursing Times* (Occasional Paper); **74**, 15; p. 60.
Hickley, M. (1978). Christian teaching concerning death — an Anglican approach *Nursing Times* (Occasional Paper); **74**, 15; pp. 59–60.
Purcell, W. (1978). *A Time to Die*. Oxford: A.R. Mowbray. (Christian Approach.)
Rabinowicz, H. (1979). The Jewish view of death. *Nursing Times;* **75**, 18; p. 757.
Richards, F. (1977). What they believe and why; Part 3, Muslims, Hindus and Buddhists. *Nursing Mirror;* **44**, 17; p. 67.

Psychosocial Aspects

McGrory, A. (1978). *A Well Model Approach to Care of the Dying Client*. New York: McGraw-Hill.
Schoenberg, B. *et al.* (1972). *Psychosocial Aspects of Terminal Care*. New York: Columbia University Press.

Personal Viewpoints

Lewis, C.S. (1961). *A Grief Observed*. London: Faber & Faber.
Smith, J–A.K. (1977). *Free Fall*. London: S.P.C.K.
Stephens, S. (1972). *Death Comes Home*. Oxford: A.R. Mowbray.

Dying Children

Burton, L. ed. (1974). *Care of the Child facing Death* London: Routledge & Kegan Paul.
Easson, W.M. (1970). *The Dying Child*. Illinois: Charles C. Thomas.
Gyulay, J.E. (1978). *The Dying Child*. New York: McGraw-Hill.

Grief and Bereavement

Dunlop, R.S. (1978). *Helping the Bereaved*. Maryland: The Charles Press.
Gorer, G. (1965). *Death, Grief and Mourning in Contemporary Britain*. London: Cresset Press.
Murray Parkes, C. (1972). *Bereavement; Studies of Grief in Adult Life*. Harmondsworth: Penguin Books.
Pett, D. (1979). Grief in hospital. *Nursing Times*; **75**, 17; pp. 709–712.
Pincus, L. (1981). *Death and the Family*. London: Faber & Faber.
Torrie, M. (1975). *Begin Again*. 2nd edn. London: J.M. Dent.

Ethics

Amulree, Lord, *et al*. (1979). *On Dying Well — An Anglican Contribution to the Debate on Euthanasia*. London: Church Information Office.
Glover, J. (1977). *Causing Death and Saving Lives*. Harmondsworth: Penguin Books.
International Work Group in Death, Dying and Bereavement (1979). Assumptions and principles underlying standards for terminal care. *Nursing Times* (Occasional Paper); **75**, 17; pp. 69–70.
Lack, S., Lamerton, R. (1974). *The Hour of Our Death*. London: Geoffrey Chapman Publishers.
Vere, D. (1971). *The Alternative to Voluntary Euthanasia*. London: Christian Medical Fellowship Publications.

Addresses:

Citizens Advice Bureau — (see local telephone directory).
Cruse (the organisation for widows and their children): Cruse House, 126 Sheen Road, Richmond, Surrey, TW9 1UR.
Exit — Euthanasia Society: 13 Prince of Wales Terrace, London, W8.
Family Welfare Association: Central Office, 501 Kingsland Road, London, E8. (Local branches in telephone directory.)
Marie Curie Memorial Foundation Homes (for patients dying of cancer): Edenhall, 11 Lyndhurst Gardens, Hampstead, London, NW3 5NS.
Multiple Sclerosis Society: 4 Tachbrook Street, London, SW1.
Society of Compassionate Friends (for parents who have lost children): National Secretary, 8 Westfield Road, Rugby, Warwickshire.
Stillbirth and Perinatal Death Association, 15a Christchurch Hill, London NW3 1JY.

Index